TOUCH THEM WITH LOVE

Phil Edwardes has been a practising healer for many years. He is the author of an earlier book, *Healing For You*, and appeared in Channel 4's TV series *The Medicine Men*.

Annette De Saulles is a freelance writer, living and working in West Sussex.

by the same author

HEALING FOR YOU

Touch Them With
LOVE

AN ACCOUNT OF

A HEALER'S WORK

AND BELIEFS

Phil Edwardes
with
Annette De Saulles

ELEMENT
Shaftesbury, Dorset ● Rockport, Massachusetts
Brisbane, Queensland

© Phil Edwardes and Annette De Saulles 1994

First published in Great Britain in 1994 by
Element Books Limited
Shaftesbury, Dorset

Published in the USA in 1994 by
Element, Inc.
42 Broadway, Rockport, MA 01966

Published in Australia by
Element Books Limited for
Jacaranda Wiley Limited,
33 Park Road, Milton, Brisbane, 4064

Cover illustration by Pictor
Cover design by Max Fairbrother
Text design by Roger Lightfoot
Typeset by Footnote Graphics, Warminster, Wiltshire
Printed and bound in Great Britain by
Redwood Books Limited, Trowbridge, Wiltshire

British Library Cataloguing in Publication
data available

Library of Congress Cataloging in publication
data available

ISBN 1–85230–555–X

Contents

Healing is real, a part of the unchanging, natural law of life that we have not yet fully understood. It is described as the power of love, channelled through the hands of a healer, involving no drugs, surgery, religious faith or ritual. There have been many cases of a rapid and dramatic return to health in those who have already exhausted all the usual orthodox medical treatments. And the hope and comfort it brings is not just for our physical selves. Healing, more importantly, can increase our awareness of the spiritual reality of our lives, our own unique potential. It can open the door to the great adventure of BEING.

But often in the world's most crowded streets
But often, in the din of strife
There rises an unspeakable desire
After the knowledge of our buried life,
A thirst to spend our fire and restless force
In tracking out our true, original course . . .

Matthew Arnold : *The Buried Life*

FOREWORD

by
Cliff Michelmore
CBE, FRSA

It is always disconcerting to have one's prejudices refuted and it is even more uncomfortable when an opinion has been held, with obstinacy, for a long time.

Ever since I can remember I have had my suspicions about the claims of healers. I have shared the antipathy of conventional medical practitioners who have, not unreasonably, wanted proof that healing really does work and is not just psychosomatic or something which works for people with imaginary ailments. In other words I suppose I was looking for evidence that it was not some form of confidence trick. My other suspicion lurked around the prefacing of the healer with the words 'spiritual' or 'faith'. What if I was neither 'spiritual' nor 'faithful'? When I went to see Phil Edwardes many of my long-standing concerns were foremost in my mind. In short I was sceptical about any chance of relief for a back pain which had persisted in spite of the attentions of doctors, surgeons, chiropractors, masseurs and osteopaths.

My own experience is much less dramatic than some you will read in this book but, nevertheless, after a short series of visits my – almost chronic – back trouble has greatly eased and I have not been back to a physiotherapist since.

Like many other people I did not know what to expect when I went to Roundstreet but, having been there, I can assure you that it was not only immensely comforting it also, in my case, was very effective in bringing relief.

You may have come to healing, as I did, hoping that there was 'something in it', or you may have come because you have tried everything else and a friend has told you about

Phil Edwardes. Whatever it is that has brought you in touch with him I assure you that at Roundstreet you have found a man who makes no claims other than he is a channel along which can flow the power of healing. As you will read in this book that power is not his but there are many who will testify to having received its benefits.

The accounts of healing contained in this book have been confirmed in signed statements by the patients named.

1

A Late Starter*

Re-examine all you have been told. Dismiss what insults
your soul.

Walt Whitman

I never really aspired to become a healer, and yet at the age
of forty-seven I became one. Although there had been signs
to this effect some twenty years earlier, I was not prepared
to recognize them for it was too much to believe that anyone
as flawed as I could possibly have this gift. I resisted until
something happened which forced me to face the reality, and
only then did I begin to understand the meaning and purpose
of my existence.

The life I led up till 1977 is hardly of significance to anyone,
but it serves to show that the designer who created us does
not discriminate when he needs a channel for his healing
love. Looking back I can see that events which at the time
I regarded as misfortunes played their part in leading me to
where I am now.

My beginnings were not quite as obscure as the character in
Oscar Wilde's play who was found 'in a handbag, at Victoria
Station', but very nearly so. I was born a bastard. I mean that
literally. It was not until I was forty-eight that I discovered the
circumstances surrounding my birth, and even then I could
not find out much, except that my mother had not wanted
me. When the baby that was to be me became due she had left
her home in Romsey and gone to London, taking a room in a

* The material in this chapter is condensed from *Healing for You*, by
Phil Edwardes and James McConnell, Thorsons, 1985.

lodging house in a Victorian terrace somewhere in Mayfair. A fortnight later she was back in Romsey. As for me, I was carted off in an open car driven by a man with red hair. And that's all I know about my arrival in the world.

My earliest memories go back to the age of three, when I was living at Yew Lodge, a big Victorian house at Havant, near Portsmouth. It was the home of Mrs Edwardes, who had taken me into her care after I was abandoned by my mother. I grew up knowing her as Mama. Her father had been an admiral in the Royal Navy and her husband Captain of HMS Canterbury, whose ship's bell now hangs in Canterbury Cathedral and is struck every day in remembrance of the men who perished at sea.

Mama had a son and daughter of her own and to supplement a meagre service pension, she boarded the children of parents whose jobs took them away from England for long periods. A small woman with a very forceful character, she lived by strict Victorian standards and ruled the herd of children by those same standards. Her discipline was firm but loving and I loved her in return.

Meals were strictly supervised and if one of us was guilty of bad manners Mama would lean forward and administer a sharp rap on the knuckles. Every Sunday we had to go to church, where Mama would sit in the row behind and give any offender a whack on the shoulder with her umbrella.

I did not resent Mama's strict regime. It was my experiences at boarding school that turned me into a rebel.

At seven years old I was sent to Emsworth House and the wrench of leaving Mama and Yew Lodge was very great. I never discovered how my education was paid for – all three schools I attended were independent, but I cannot say that the money was well spent.

From my memories of Emsworth House one stands out vividly: I was in the common room with a number of other boys one day. No doubt we were fooling about but I was not conscious of doing anything bad. Suddenly a master appeared and, sweeping through the room, he picked on me and grabbed me by the scruff of the neck. He took me into the next room, made me bend over and gave me a thrashing with a cane. It was a very painful and unpleasant experience. I never knew what my offence had been, but that was probably the moment when the spirit of rebellion was born in me.

In 1939, aged nine, I went on to Fernden School and for the first time I became aware what a social stigma it was to be illegitimate. Somehow the other boys had found out about it and they were very cruel in their mockery.

The insults continued when I went on to Sherborne in Dorset. I know it is one of the best public schools but the war was on and standards had gone down. By now I was a confirmed rebel and rules meant little to me, so I was always coming up against the system. I had little enthusiasm for organized team games and absolutely no ambition to get into the sixth form. It was made very clear to me that there was something unacceptable about me.

'Edwardes', one master said, 'you'll end up as a crossing-sweeper, that's all you're good for.'

Looking back on my public school days, I think that what scarred me most was the religious teaching and the sermons in chapel. The Divinity classes reinforced my feeling that I was a lost cause, the sermons leading me to believe that I myself was the product of wickedness and vice – having been born illegitimate. If all these preachings were true I had precious little hope in this world and a damn sight less in the world to come.

But there are always two sides to a coin. My instinct told me that all this talk of damnation and hell-fire could not be right and in a way this is what saved me, for my rejection of the accepted doctrines led me to do my own questioning. I set out to try and discover for myself about such fundamental matters as the nature of the creation, the purpose of human existence and man's relationship with the deity.

When at last I was free of school it was 1946 and National Service was still in operation. The armed forces with their

regimentation were not for me, so I joined the Palestine Police
and spent most of my eighteen months as an armed constable
patrolling the docks at Haifa.

Back in England in 1948, I applied for a job with the
Metropolitan Police and actually passed the entrance exam.
But in the meantime the Palestine Police Resettlement Officer
had got me a job in the Rhodesian Police. However, the
tedious paperwork and petty rules brought out the rebel in
me and I left after a short time.

My next job was on the railway that ran from Northern to
Southern Rhodesia. I enjoyed that time of my life and had a
lot of fun. The work was hard but the food was good and I
slept like a log. The pay was generous and even as a trainee
fireman I had an African servant. That way I earned the only
qualification I possess: I ended up as a fully qualified Railway
Steam Locomotive Fireman.

My behaviour, however, was too riotous for the railway
company and they gave me the sack. I'm afraid that's the
kind of fellow I was in those days.

I then took a job as a bus driver in Salisbury, the capital
of Southern Rhodesia (now Zimbabwe), but this only lasted
six months. After five accidents in four months, I was asked,
not unreasonably, to resign.

After a spell as a meter reader for the electricity company,
I joined up with a friend and we went out to live rough
in the bush. Under the stars I had a chance to think. I
was twenty-one, my life seemed aimless and I was getting
nowhere, so I decided to return home to England.

But I continued to drift from job to job until, in 1959,
an incident occurred which made a big impression on me.
It stood out from the negative aspect of my life at that time
as something positive and worthwhile.

I was walking beside a lake near Kineton in Warwickshire
when I noticed something floating in the water about thirty
yards out. It was a woman, alive, but making no attempt to
swim. It was lucky I was a strong swimmer. That woman did
not want to be rescued – she fought me desperately and even
when I had finally managed to bring her to shore, she tried to

throw herself back into the water. I had to restrain her until help arrived.

I visited her later in hospital and learned that it was the loneliness of bereavement that had led her to such a desperate action. Since her husband's death she could see no purpose in going on living. All the same she was grateful. It had been an impulsive action and she was glad I'd come along and hauled her out. She must have made a good story of it because some time later I received an Honorary Testimonial, on vellum, from the Royal Humane Society. It was something to add to my certificate as a Railway Steam Locomotive Fireman.

In 1960 I met Ann, who was soon to become my wife. Then, through a friend, I was lucky enough to get the tenancy of a garage and service station in a small village in Sussex. The business prospered and by 1967 we were able to acquire the lease of a garage near Gatwick Airport and another at Chessington.

When Roundstreet House came on the market I knew at once that it was the place for me. The oldest part of the house dated back to Tudor times. Opposite the front door was an old coach-house and the whole property was surrounded by a beautiful rose garden. At last my life seemed to have settled down into an organized pattern. My family were delighted to be living in the country, and business was booming.

Then an event occurred which changed everything.

Phillip, my second son, really thrived on this new life. At the age of nine he was two years ahead of his contemporaries at school. And this was not only in academic work. He came out as *victor ludorum* competing against boys of thirteen. Amongst his group he was the natural leader and perhaps this was the reason for the touch of arrogance which was his only fault.

Across the road from our house is a minor road that leads down to a few farms and houses. Beyond a cattle grid there is a winding hill where an old oak stands. On a summer's day in 1970 Phillip and some friends went cycling down this track. As usual Phillip was in the lead, head down to reduce wind resistance. The tractor coming up the hill was being driven by an elderly learner-driver. In a mistaken effort to avoid the boys he drove across the track onto the grass verge on the right-hand side. Phillip's head struck the tractor, now careering out of control, and before the old man could stop it, a back and a front wheel ran over his chest.

Philip was still lying unconscious on the track when I reached the spot. The sight of him was a terrible and unforgettable shock. He was rushed to hospital in Guildford and taken into intensive care, where he was X-rayed and examined by two doctors. He had suffered extensive brain damage and severe internal injuries. Neither of the doctors thought that he could live and all that we could do now was wait.

Although I was shattered by this news I personally did not give up hope. And at this point I must forewarn the reader that what follows may be difficult to believe, but I am only relating what happened, exactly as it happened and as I experienced it.

Though not a spiritualist myself I had been in contact with spiritualists during the early years of my marriage to Ann when we were living in Banbury. I had also made friends with some spiritual healers who lived in Oxford. When I'd heard what the doctors had to say I immediately telephoned these friends in Oxford. I told them about what had happened to Phillip and described his present condition. I asked them to give him absent healing – sometimes known as distant healing.

All that night I sat by the bedside of my unconscious son. In the early hours he vomited a little dried blood. When the same doctors came in the morning they seemed surprised that he was still alive and further X-rays were taken with a portable machine. The doctors were puzzled. An hour later they returned and took another X-ray – the internal injuries had disappeared overnight! The only signs of damage now were the large bruised areas on his arms and shoulders and the scoring of the flesh on his chest. The doctors were at a loss to account for his amazing recovery. I knew that this was the power of absent healing, but I kept my counsel.

Phillip did not regain consciousness for three weeks. During that period my friends in Oxford continued to direct absent healing to him. When at last he did come round, Phillip was far from normal. The personality which emerged from the long coma was changed and one felt that he had brought back with him the atmosphere of a very beautiful place.

When he returned home he had to learn to walk all over again and learn to ride a bike from scratch. Whereas before he had been inclined to arrogance he was now very sensitive to other people's moods. And he could not bear conflict of any kind, for instance the sound of other children squabbling.

Ann and I would not accept the fact that his brain damage was permanent – we were sure that he'd become normal again. But it took a long time, years, and as there was no school that he could fit into, he went from one to another. He had forgotten all about the rules and regulations of a school and it was not exactly helpful that he showed no respect at all for the masters. During classes he would get up and wander about, or go and talk to the lady who cleaned the school. In a way he was living in another world, but with it all he was a lovable and loving person. By the age of sixteen 'Gentle Phil', as he was called, was holding down a minor job in a factory nearby.

But that's looking ahead. There was further unhappiness in the intervening years. It is never easy to talk about the failure of a marriage – the reasons are always too complex and intimate to be shared with the outside world. All I want to say is that after ten years of marriage it had become obvious that Ann and I were incompatible. We were slowly destroying each other and there was only one solution to the increasing unhappiness and stress. We agreed to separate, though Ann continued to play an important role in the life of the children.

There was another big gap in my life. On my thirty-fifth birthday I had lost Mama, the one person in the world whom I could look on as a parent. She died on 25th October 1965. The loss of her affected me keenly and during the years that followed I began to feel more and more a need to know something about the family I'd sprung from. I wanted to clear up the question of my parentage and birth. It is strange how much a thing like that can matter, but it's a deep human need to know by whose agency you came into the world and until you find out, you have a sense that somehow you don't belong.

I was already into my forties when I at last decided to do something about it.

Mama had explained to me, as soon as I was old enough to understand, that I was not really her son. I'd often asked her who I really was, who were my parents, why my family had not wanted me. The questions seemed to upset her, and I could not understand why she always avoided them. I sensed some mystery there.

The Salvation Army has a department in London for tracing people, especially the parents of children who have lost touch with their families. They have a lot of resources and plenty of experience and they provide the service free, so I started off by going to them.

It took them a little time but eventually they let me know that they had succeeded in tracing my mother. For some reason they would not tell me who she was or where to find her. Here was another mystery.

Biding my time, I started to put money into a savings fund. When I had enough I engaged a private detective agency to take up the search, and after a couple of months they reported to me that they had found the register of my birth at Somerset House. My father's surname had been entered as Seymour, the name I'd been given when I first went to Yew Lodge. It turned out to be false. My grandfather's name was Stride. The agency had been able to trace my mother's last known address, at a place called Nursling Mill, near Romsey in Hampshire.

I was at Barwell Motors in Chessington when I heard the news — I jumped straight into a car and drove down to Romsey, where I was able to locate the site of Nursling Mill. It was on the Test to the east of Romsey, just outside the town. But the mill itself had vanished, long since abandoned.

Tramping the fields in my business suit I met a farmer

who had worked in the neighbourhood since a boy. Yes, he remembered Nursling Mill and the woman who had lived there. And he'd known of the Strides, a well-off family with a house on the Test and a fine stretch of fishing. There were two daughters, he remembered, good-looking girls. The woman who had lived at the Mill – my mother – had married a solicitor in Romsey, name of Swayne, and when old man Stride died she'd inherited half his fortune. There'd been a son, Henry, by that marriage – who would be ten years older than me. As to other children, he didn't know. He had not seen Mrs Swayne for years but he'd heard that she was still living in Romsey – and it so happened that he knew the address.

It turned out to be a detached house on the outskirts of the town. I felt both nervous and excited as I stood on the doorstep waiting for my knock to be answered. In a few minutes I'd be looking at the mother who had brought me into the world.

The door was opened by a woman who could not have been more than fifty – not nearly old enough to have been my mother. Her look of surprise quickly changed. She stared at me as if she thought she must have met me somewhere.

'My name's Edwardes,' I said. 'Could I have a few words with the lady who lives here – an elderly lady?'

I hoped that the briefcase I was carrying would support my story that I had some business to discuss with the 'elderly lady'. But my cover was already blown.

'I know who you are', she said, in a voice that was not unfriendly. 'You're Henry's younger brother – aren't you?'

'Yes,' I admitted.

'He's often wondered what became of you.' She was still studying my face. 'You're very like him, you know.'

'Are you . . . ?' I started, wondering if this woman could be a sister of mine.

'Oh, I'm sorry! I should have explained. I'm Beth, Henry's wife. Come in and I'll phone Henry. He works in Romsey.'

It took Henry less than ten minutes to hurry back from his office. His appearance provided a rough specification of what I could expect to look like in ten years' time.

The conversation which followed was a curious one, to say the least, but at last I steered it round to the subject of my mother.

She was in a downstairs room, Beth told me. I caught the look she exchanged with Henry and realized that the subject was painful to them.

'Could I see her?'

Again that quick exchange of glances.

'She's very old, you understand', Henry said. 'Her mind's gone. I don't think she'll recognize you – even if she remembers anything about you.'

'I'd still like to see her.'

Beth led me down a passage, opened a door and left me to go in on my own. Entering the bedroom I had a strong sense of unreality. This was the moment I had been looking forward to for so long and now that it had come my feelings were frozen.

The room was dark and close. It was obvious that the woman in the bed was in the early stages of senile decay. The eyes that turned towards me were blank and disinterested. I could feel neither resentment nor tenderness towards her. But I very badly wanted her to know who I was.

'I'm your son,' I said. There was no other clue I could give her, for at that time I still knew nothing about the circumstances of my birth. 'Do you remember – forty years ago?'

It meant nothing to her. Talking to her was very difficult and it took me a long time to get anything through to her. In the end she seemed to realize vaguely who I was, but about my father she could tell me nothing. Her mind wandered away and further conversation became pointless, so I left her to her ramblings and quietly closed the door. I never saw her again.

From my half-brother I learned that my father had owned a garage in Southampton – an odd coincidence. He did not know anything more about him, but he was able to tell me that just before my birth my mother had gone up to London for a couple of weeks. 'Mummy is sick', he had been told. Her secrecy was understandable since Henry's father was not my father and not till years later did she tell him that he had a half-brother somewhere in the world.

From Henry I learned that I had a sister, a real sister with the same mother and father. Her name was Pam and she lived with her husband and four children in Southend.

That information made the whole quest worthwhile.

It was some days before I was able to drive to Southend. Pam lived in a terraced house with a small garden. The door was opened by a lovely young woman ten years younger than me.

I said 'Are you Pam?'

'Yes.'

'I'm your brother.'

There had been no feelings when I saw my mother but this meeting was deeply emotional, at the same time painful and thrilling. At last I had found someone to whom I really belonged through blood ties. It may be hard for those who have always had the security of a family background to understand how much this meant. Though we were strangers we quickly found that we had great affinity and that we saw things in the same way. Pam had a warm-hearted approach to people and I found I could respond to her open personality.

Later she and her family moved quite near to us in Sussex. Pam was a trained nurse and got a job as matron of a nursing home there. We were able to see a lot of each other and our relationship grew deeper and deeper. We never made any effort to trace our father – there seemed little point and, besides, the garage he owned, as well as the municipal records, had gone up in the blitz during World War II. Nor could she tell me any more than Henry had about the mystery of my 'adoption' by Mama and the funding of my education.

When, some time later, we heard that our mother had died, we felt no real grief. The important thing was that late in life we had each found kith and kin – she a brother and I a sister.

The Gatwick Airport garage was now so profitable that I had given up both the other garages to concentrate my efforts on the off-airport parking business. At that time the volume of traffic at Gatwick was building up and we were in great demand from travellers who wanted their cars garaged while they were abroad. We would take them to Departure and pick them up at Arrival when they returned. Many of them wanted their cars serviced or repaired during their absence. We provided a twenty-four hour service and gruelling work it was – a short week was 80 hours and on some weeks I was working up to 120 hours. There were days when I did not get home till two in the morning and was off again at seven.

My right-hand person in this mammoth task was Sue, a young woman of about twenty who had worked for me since my first garage tenancy. She was a glutton for work, not only doing the books but driving the mini-bus, selling petrol, dealing with the staff and their pay, cleaning the lavatories – you name it.

Working so closely with Sue I came to appreciate her marvellous qualities. Having recently been through the painful experience of a failed marriage I was hesitant about entering into any new commitment, but as time went on I realized that I had at last found the perfect partner. We became engaged, and in due course married. So Sue came to fill the gap left at Roundstreet House by the departure of Ann.

It was really thanks to an initiative of Sue's that something happened which caused me to completely change my way of life.

I had for a long time been interested in the paranormal. In the days when I was living and working in Banbury I had been a member of a discussion group. We were not irresponsible dabblers in the occult but serious and dedicated people in search of knowledge and understanding. When I moved to Newbury another group used to meet in my flat to discuss paranormal subjects. One of its members was Percy Corbett, who later became secretary of the Church's Fellowship for Psychic and Spiritual Studies.

I was sitting one evening in my favourite chair with the others round me. It's an old craftsman-built wooden chair with a high back and arm-rests and it stands today in the healing room at Roundstreet. All at once I felt as if an electric current were pulsing down my arms. The power seemed to originate somewhere behind me and my hands were tingling so much that it would not have surprised me to see sparks coming from the tips of my fingers.

I told the others what I was feeling and we all joined hands to see what would happen. Immediately they all felt the same thing, like an electric charge going through their bodies.

Even Percy Corbett could not account for this and it did not occur to any of them that it might be connected with a healing power – certainly not to me. I knew that there were healers but I assumed they must be people of high character who led blameless lives. Not someone born a bastard, whose only qualification was as a Railway Steam Locomotive Fireman.

Nonetheless, experiences like that increased my interest in things beyond the normal and in the years that followed I had contact with a number of sensitives – or mediums, as they are sometimes called. Some very strange things happened, but this is a book about healing and not spiritualism, so I will only say that they altered my views on such fundamental things as life and death. I now had evidence that physical death did not extinguish life so, I reasoned, there must be some purpose in living. The religious teaching at school had led me to associate God with judgement, damnation and hell-fire, but now I had become convinced that, in spite of appearances to the contrary, a loving design lies behind human and cosmic existence. This implied a loving designer. The word 'God' was for me bound up with doctrines I could not accept, which is why I prefer to speak of the creator spirit as 'the Guv'nor'. Not till many years had passed was I to realize that I had a part to play in His grand design.

During my early days as a garage manager I had been given an indication that I might have a healing power, but I still shied away from it. At one of the garages where I worked there was a regular customer by the name of Charlie Woods – 'Timbers'. He would drop in for a cup of tea and we'd often sit and chat about the ways of the world and his problems with his duodenum.

One day he came in clasping his belly and grimacing with pain. 'God, my stomach's killing me!' he complained.

'Something disagree with you, Timbers?'

'No, I'm getting it all the time now. Can't keep anything down. I can't sleep at night and my stomach's so sore I can't even bear to touch it. It's them ulcers. My doctor's given me pills, ought to make it better but they don't do any good.'

While he was talking I felt heat in my hands. I had experienced this before but had not connected it with any healing power. I said quite casually, 'Have you thought of going to a healer like Harry Edwards? He has a big house near Guildford where people go to be healed.'

'Edwards? Any relation of yours?'

'No. We spell our names differently. He's healed a lot of people.'

'A healer? No, I never thought of that. What's a healer do?'

The heat was still in my hands but I did not want to say anything about that. I certainly was not going to claim that I had any healing power in me. All the same I felt I wanted to do something about Charlie Woods.

I said, 'Sometimes the healer has to put his hands on you – like this. Put your hand on the table, Timbers.'

He put his hand on the table and I held my own about twelve inches over it. 'Can you feel anything?' I asked.

'Your hands! They're hot!'

'That's healing,' I said and went on to talk about something else.

Charlie Woods was amazed but at the time neither of us put great significance on it. You'd expect healing to be carried out in a church or somewhere by a man in a white surplice, not by a garage manager in the dingy little office at the back of the workshop. Charlie went on his way and I forgot all about it.

Three weeks later he turned up again, this time a different man. His face was cheerful and smiling and he was thumping his stomach as he came in.

'I don't know what you did, Phil, but you cured the trouble.'

My mind was on automobile repairs and I did not immediately grasp what he meant.

'My stomach!' he said. 'You did the trick. The pain's gone and I'm sleeping nights. I can eat what I like now. Had a steak last night and it went down a treat. None of those pains that used to nearly kill me.'

Stomach ulcers, even I knew this, are often caused by worry and stress, sometimes anxiety or fear. Perhaps something else had occurred to take a load off Timbers' mind, but I did not really think that I was responsible.

Later I had more direct evidence and I might have acted on it if I had not received what seemed like a rebuff.

Some time before, I had got to know a young lad of sixteen who suffered from very severe curvature of the spine. It was really double curvature because his spine was bent in an S-shape, and locked in that position. There was a hump where his spine went behind one shoulder-blade, and he had to get about on crutches because his legs were withered. As orthodox treatment was not helping, I pursuaded him to let me take him to see Harry Edwards.

Harry Edwards sat him on a low, square stool and called me over. He made me put my hand on the injured part of my friend's back, before putting his own hand over mine. I felt the boy's vertebrae move under my hand. He stood up straightened. The hump had gone. He was not able to walk out of there without his crutches but from that day forward his spine was straight. Oddly, he never went back for more healing.

Back at home I wrote to Harry Edwards to tell him what I had experienced, but I never received a reply.

Early in the summer of 1977 Sue and I were having lunch at a pub not far from home. Sue began to chat to the woman behind the food bar. She was interested in the practice of yoga but some problems had cropped up which were troubling. Sue invited her to call at our house for a talk, thinking that perhaps I could be of some help to her.

The following Sunday she arrived with a friend whom she introduced as Maria. We were in the sitting room discussing the problem when Sue noticed that Maria was sitting on the edge of the sofa, very uncomfortable and awkward.

'It's this allergy,' Maria explained, and thereupon she turned her back and pulled up her T-shirt. The lower part of her back was in a terrible state, which I can only describe as like raw steak.

She explained that her doctor had not yet discovered what was causing the allergy, so she was not receiving treatment for it.

Looking at her back I began to feel the odd sensation in my hands which I now associate with healing – a kind of trembling and tingling plus a feeling of heat. I wanted to touch Maria's back.

I got up and asked her to keep still while I placed my fingertips on the small of her back. I could feel the healing pouring through my hands. It lasted for several seconds.

'What's happening?' Maria asked.

'I think you're getting some healing. Just keep still.'

'What's healing?'

'Never mind.'

She kept still and waited. My fingers were shaking slightly but I hardly touched her back. Later she told me that during those moments she had an extraordinary sensation, 'as if my whole inside was being shaken up'. When the healing sensation stopped I went back to my seat.

By next morning all Maria's pain had gone and the rawness was healed. Her skin was flaky as if recovering from sunburn and soon it was completely back to normal.

After the incident with Maria I made up my mind to go and see a healer named M. H. Tester who lived a few miles away. I had read his book and knew his reputation. He gave me an appointment and I went to see him. He listened in silence to what I told him.

'Phil, you're a healer,' he said. 'Get on with it.'

Tester's words gave me the push I needed but it was largely

due to Sue's encouragement that I decided to give it a try. I had put it off for long enough and, looking back, I sometimes wonder if I wasted twenty years of my life. But perhaps the Guv'nor knew I was not ready to start working for him till now. It was only recently that I had discovered about my roots and had at last found a sister who was blood of my blood. And I now had as a helpmate someone who understood what sort of person I really was and supported me completely.

Though the Gatwick operation was booming it gave me no real satisfaction. I was restless, and for some time had had a strong feeling that there was something else I ought to be doing. Sue assured me she could handle the business if I came in for one day a week – she was already responsible for everything except the repairs side, which I handled, and someone else could take that on.

We agreed to try it for a year. If I turned out to be no good as a healer I'd go back to the garage.

Word soon got around that there was a healer at Round-street Common and people began to come for treatment. But it was building up only slowly. A friend acting on my behalf persuaded me to let her book a nearby town hall so that I could give a talk on healing and she advertised it in the local paper. I'd never spoken in public before and I found the 'lecture' part very difficult. It all became much easier when we moved on to 'questions' and I began to get some feedback from my audience. Even years later new patients often told me they had been to that lecture.

With the gradual increase in patients, accommodation became a problem. To begin with I had done my healing in the old Tudor part of the main house. A flight of steps led up from my study to a small room or landing under the eaves and I used this as a healing room, although it was far from ideal. Some patients could not manage the stairs and I was very much on top of the life of the house.

Opposite the front door was the coach-house, which I'd had plans for for some time. I was sure it could be adapted to provide a waiting room and a healing room. The improvements and refurbishing would cost a bit of money, so I made an appointment to see my bank manager.

He received me in his private office and was very friendly and affable until I told him that I wanted to borrow £3,000 – then his eyebrows went up. 'Well, I'm not sure that we can help you there, Mr Edwardes,' he said.

'But I've been a customer of yours for fifteen years and you've lent me money before.'

'Yes, I appreciate that, but things were different then. You don't have a regular job any more, do you?'

'No.'

'What security can you offer?'

'None, I'm afraid. That's why I need the loan.'

He pursed his lips and looked very dubious. It so happened that I had in my briefcase a copy of *Psychic News* which contained an article about some of my patients and how they had been healed. On an impulse I took it out and handed it to him, folded at the place.

He put on his glasses and read it through. Then he looked at me thoughtfully. 'Do you know, I once went to a healer in Surrey. His name was Harry Edwards. I had trouble with my hip and the doctors were getting nowhere with it, but Harry Edwards healed it. I've never had any trouble with it since.'

I said, 'Perhaps you can see from that article that I work for the Guv'nor, too.'

'Yes,' he agreed with a smile. 'I think you do.'

'Well, where,' I asked him, 'could you get a better reference for a loan?'

With the bank's £3,000 behind me I was able to put the necessary alterations in hand straight away. I did the work myself, laying bricks, building a chimney stack of which I am not very proud, fixing guttering, putting a pine ceiling in the healing room. Sue had already given birth to our third son and was still having to run the garage. Without her pay we had not enough to live on.

'Don't worry,' we'd been told. 'Sue will be at home before the baby is toddling.'

Amongst her many activities at the garage, Sue always organized a little syndicate of eight that put in an entry every week for Littlewood's Football Pool. One day in September she was sitting at her desk which commanded a view of the forecourt when she saw a man park his car and get out. He was wearing a business suit and carrying a briefcase. She thought he looked just like the kind of official who comes round to inspect the toilet facilities or the VAT records, so when he came into her office she received him warily.

'You are Susan Edwardes of Salford's Garage, Gatwick?' he asked.

'That's right.'

'I've come to inform you that you have won the top prize in Littlewood's Football Pool.'

It was obviously some sort of spoof, so Sue kept up the game. 'Oh, yes. How much for?'

'£750,000.'

It took him all of five minutes to convince her that this was no joke. *We had won the Pools!*

Of course, the prize had to be divided into eight, the number of people in the syndicate. One of the eight was a girl who had actually left her job at the garage the previous week, but Sue had paid her share for her and included her in the syndicate this one last time. Even the girl did not know that she was 'in', but Sue, typically, insisted that she must be included in the winnings. It came to £93,750 each.

We had to go up to London for the ceremonial presentation of the enormous cheque by Littlewoods, though it was actually handed over to us by the comedians Little and Large. The photographers were more interested in the celebrated comics than in the eight grinning winners from Salford's Garage.

There were lots of lads there from the City to tell us how to invest our money. I had already been warned 'Don't accept anything less than 17 per cent' – which made me a little wary of the representative of a well-known High Street bank who came to Roundstreet and told me that as a special gesture he could get me 8 per cent.

This windfall made all the difference to us. With the income from our capital we had enough to live on and Sue was able to give up her job at the garage and be at home all the time – just as Toby started toddling.

Most satisfactory of all, I was able to repay the loan the bank manager had granted me and prove to him that his confidence in my credit-worthiness had not been misplaced.

There had been no doubt in my mind about what this manna from heaven was to be used for. It provided us with independent means so that I could continue to work as a healer and Sue could fulfil her role as mother and housewife. Being unearned income, the revenue attracted a higher rate of tax and my net income was now at a very basic level. Just then interest rates were high, but when they fell a couple of years later, our income was much reduced.

People sometimes judge a healer by the kind of life he leads. Many expect that, because he is exercising a God-given gift, he should adopt a life of penury and self-denial, not only for himself but for his family as well. Contrary to popular belief, a healer is not someone special – he is a human being like anybody else. It is true that the more genuinely caring he is about those who come to him for help, the more effective his healing will be. If he was so self-centred that his aim in life was to amass material possessions it is unlikely that he would make a good healer. Some critics argue that a true healer should make no monetary charge for his or her services. My response to these critics is that if a healer has given up all other means of income so that he can be of service to others, it is only proper that he should receive something with which he can support himself and his family.

I live a simple life with few luxuries but I do not fast or perform arduous religious exercises. I enjoy life and the good things of this earth. If the Guv'nor did not intend us to enjoy his creation why did he make it so beautiful and provide us with the senses to appreciate it? Since I became a healer my

life and outlook have of course changed, but I am in no sense
an ascetic and am certainly not anyone's idea of a guru or
holy man.

With Sue at home and attending to the everyday demands
of a growing family, I had a much more favourable background for my healing. Work on the coach-house was at last
completed and the flow of patients was steadily increasing.
The people who came or were brought to see me had nothing
in common except that they were all ailing in one way or
another. There was tremendous variation in the type of illness
for which they were seeking help, and also in their attitudes
towards healing. Almost without exception they were cases
where orthodox medicine had failed. Many had already tried
other forms of complementary medicine – homoeopathy,
hypnotism or acupuncture.

They had come to me as a last resort.

The general public's growing awareness of what is sometimes
referred to as alternative medicine led Anglia Television to
prepare a series of documentary films on the subject during
1980-81. The title of the series was *The Medicine Men*,
and there was also to be a book based on it. Each of
the eight weekly programmes was to feature one of the
complementary forms of medicine. Healing was fifth on
the list.

The TV crew came down for a day's filming at Roundstreet
and the series was shown in the early months of 1982. Our
reward was a brief shot of me in the healing room with one
of my patients.

The showing of this film had good results, as a number of
patients who came to me subsequently said that seeing *The
Medicine Men* or reading the book had made them decide to
give healing a try.

During my seventeen years as a healer I have seen nearly
five thousand patients. That may seem few compared with
the hundreds of thousands of a Harry Edwards, a Don
Greenbank or a Tom Pilgrim. Each healer has his own style

and mine involves giving each patient a lot of time and, when necessary, seeing them over a long period.

During those seventeen years I have come to understand better how healing works and how I can best fulfil my part in the process. In the next chapter I will try to explain, in simple language, what healing is.

2

What Is Healing?

Do you need Me? I AM there.
You cannot see Me, yet I AM the Light you see by.
You cannot hear Me, yet I speak through your
voice.
You cannot feel Me, yet I AM the Power at work
in your hands.

from *I Am There* by J.D. Freeman

My aim in writing this book is to explain healing in a simple, factual way so that people might both be comforted to know that healing is available to them and also encouraged to investigate for themselves the message that it carries.

What is healing? I will try to describe something which may make it easier for those with a practical turn of mind to understand. When a piano tuner strikes his A fork it vibrates at 440 cycles per second. If the piano's A string above middle C is in tune, that is to say at the right combination of length and tension, it too will start resonating or vibrating in response to the sound waves emitted by the fork. If there is another piano in the room and somebody's foot is on the sustaining pedal its A string will also start to vibrate. The important thing about this process is that *energy is transferred*. When two elements are in vibrational harmony energy can pass from one to the other even if the frequencies are different. For instance, a loud A will cause audible vibrations on the A string in the next octave, which vibrates at 880 cycles per second or twice as fast.

Not only vibrating piano strings respond to external cyclic stimuli. So do people. There is of course a greater range of sound than the human ear is capable of catching. In the practice of healing there is often much vibration running through the healer or in his hands, and this is felt by the patient. These vibrations have been described as corrective in that they restore harmony. The character of these vibrations differs to suit the different needs of each patient, and even with the same patient it may differ from one session to another.

The healing vibrations are not sound vibrations but are nonetheless energy or power being *intelligently* transmitted through the healer. The healer has little or no knowledge of what needs to be done to bring about the physical changes required for the particular ailment to be healed.

That is a practical analogy which throws some light on the outward and physical signs of what is an inward and spiritual happening. An effective healer must develop a true understanding of love, and he must listen to the spiritual teaching available, to the instructions from within. This state has to be achieved by first divesting oneself of preconceived ideas and prejudices and remembering simply that God is love and that we are all part of Him and of one another. I am given help in many different ways. The Guv'nor has many messengers. In some religions they are called 'angels', which means the same thing. That is why at week-ends I sometimes seek guidance in my work by sitting quietly with a group of chosen friends waiting receptively for any messages that may come. A healer needs to know that he has this support.

One cannot be a healer without becoming intimately aware of the loving designer who created us and who cares so deeply about us. His love is the most powerful force there is and healing is love itself in action. It is effective design at work.

As Edgar Cayce, the American healer, said 'The spirit is the life, the mind is the builder and the body is the result.' Where there is harmony between spirit, mind and body you have real health. Disease occurs when that harmony is broken.

Broken it often is by the process of living. You have only to look at the ravages of time on the faces of some people to have proof that living is stressful. Yet the greater the stress the greater the chance to learn. Illness, or bereavement, or the approach of death provide an opportunity for learning in greater depth. Healing is indeed wonderful in itself but it is a pointer to even bigger things. We must look not just at the fact of healing but seek to understand also the purpose of healing.

What is healing? What is its purpose? To those two questions there is one answer: healing is evidence of the great spirit's love.

> The healing power passes from the Great Spirit through the healer's spirit to the spirit of the patient. Within the patient it takes the route SPIRIT – MIND – BODY.
> Thus the healing passes from spirit through spirit to spirit and is reflected in mind and body.

Comprehending this evidence of the Great Spirit's love is more important than a physical cure. For many the experience of healing is a turning-point in their lives. It points them in a new direction. That direct contact with the power and the glory may for some be cataclysmic.

One patient told me that, when she came for healing, it was the first time in her life she could begin to see a purpose and reason for living. Until then everything had seemed fairly hopeless. 'It totally changed my life' – a reaction echoed by many who had hoped for no more than a physical easement. Beneficial physical change is often only the beginning of healing; the implications of the healing power can change a person's direction of thought and their assumptions about life itself*.

A woman in her sixties was suffering with severe pain in her left foot and ankle. She was also a diabetic. Healing was not only successful in relieving her physical pain and easing the diabetes so that doctors could cut down her insulin intake,

---

* The material from the start of the chapter to here is condensed from *Healing for You* by Phil Edwardes and James McConnell, Thorsons, 1985.

but she also found she began to feel differently about life. She was able to relax, despite many family problems, and a colleague remarked 'I don't know what has happened to you, but you seem so serene'. Her family noticed the change too. She felt that healing had done so much for her because she had been open to it.

The first thing about healing is that there is nothing new about it. It happens all over the world under all sorts of different 'umbrellas', and always has done. Quite often those holding a particular 'umbrella' are inclined to think that healing occurs because of their 'umbrella'. This is about as sensible as supposing that umbrellas make it rain. The consequence is that there are many different prefixes attached to the word *healing*: faith healing, spiritual healing and many more – which can be confusing and indeed can put some people off. Healing does not depend upon faith, although an acceptance of the possibility of healing may help. All you really need is hope.

The second thing about healing is that the healer does not *do* any healing. He is merely a channel for something that occurs through him – in spite of the healer rather than because of him.

When healing occurs it is clear to me that I have no understanding of the detail of a particular ailment. I would not know how to start to deal with it. I say this because of all the wonderful things that have happened here through healing, and I am sure that I do not know how to bring them about.

Deirdre Faccenda did not think healing would be able to help, but was in despair after eighteen years of sickness and violent indigestion following the birth of her son. It had got so bad she could hardly go out. Doctors had been unable to find the cause, and I of course could not know either. But healing in this case was immediate and lasting.

Later, when Deirdre's mother came for treatment for her migraines, she did not think to mention the ear-ache she had suffered with constantly since she was a baby. It was only when the ear-ache abruptly stopped soon afterwards that she realized what living without pain could be like. Without my knowing of the complaint, healing had nevertheless occurred. The migraines also lessened.

Janis Moore did not mention an embarrassing skin complaint that she had suffered from for six years when she came for healing for severe migraines. She was due to go on holiday to Florida and was dreading the flight, coping with her baby son and the inevitable blinding headache. The migraines cleared up afterwards – and so did the uncomfortable sores on her buttocks and backs of her thighs that she had not mentioned. By the time Janis got back from her holiday there was now only one sore left, and this soon vanished.

Healing comes from beyond us, and to my knowledge has never hurt anyone. It must therefore come from a very loving and marvellously intelligent source.

So here at Roundstreet House it is *healing* plain and simple – without 'labels'.

Healing can restore hope – and therefore a helpfully positive approach – when it is realized that even long-standing problems, where the patient has been told by the medical profession there is nothing more that can be done, begin to show improvement.

One of my patients had suffered a serious motor cycle accident in his late teens, leaving him with various injuries and scars down one side of his body. The posterior cruciate ligament in his left knee was stretched so that the knee was not held in place properly, and by the time I saw him the damage was beginning to cause increasing problems. The orthopaedic surgeon had told him it was the oldest looking knee he had seen and that it was gradually wearing itself away. An X-ray showed a sliver of bone that had broken away. He was offered a risky 'last-resort' knee joint replacement operation, but was told that if anything went wrong, it left no choice but to amputate.

It was his osteopath who suggested my patient should come for healing as he himself had been helped by it, and my patient came along with an open mind.

With regular visits, things slowly began to improve and my

patient could move about more easily on the knee. Six months later, another orthopaedic surgeon was comparing X-rays of the knee. 'You have some new bone growing here,' he said. 'I don't know where that's come from.' And the loose sliver of bone had joined itself back on, a faint line indicating where it had rejoined.

My patient had also been left with an unpleasant and unnatural-looking scar on his left elbow. After healing, the scar tissue became smooth and resumed a normal colour – some twenty-eight years after the accident that had caused it.

The essence of healing is not just to be physically healed but to 'Know thyself'; that is, to come to the realization that you are not your body, that there is no limit to YOU. I would consider healing a failure if a person did not embark consciously on their own spiritual journey, even if physically cured. And of course, spirituality has nothing to do with being religious! Religious instruction is only what others think and teach – no religious dogma can apply to everyone. No-one has the monopoly on truth – the truth is within ourselves. Consider all the religions of the world – and then think for yourself. That is the only way to find the right path.

'. . . seek and ye shall find; knock and it shall be opened unto you.' I have done both throughout my life, which is why I am a healer. The medical profession may dismiss healing as 'psychosomatic' or 'spontaneous remission' – a comfortable tag which discourages further questioning. The religious escape from awkward questions is 'Have faith, we are not supposed to know' – but I think that man-made church dogma has done much to obscure what the great healer, Jesus Christ, meant to convey by His life and sayings. A man must base his belief on his own experience, then he *knows* rather than believes, though he can never know it all – I have my convictions but I am still searching for truth. I am sure that we are not judged by our performance on earth by some unforgiving God – life is not a test but simply a means of learning. There is a natural law of cause and effect.

A woman of seventy had been afraid for a long time of

coming to me, although in pain, because her Methodist religion would not have approved of it. Yet God (or the Guv'nor as I prefer to say) is all, therefore all is God. God is love, therefore love is God. Healing power is life force and can only be exercised with compassion, which is a part of love. Man has an urge to label everything – to make divisions where there are none. This encourages us to see differences where there are none. We ignore and disassociate ourselves from our fellow human beings, sheltering behind imaginery lines. Healing does not require the prefix 'faith' or 'spiritual', 'hand' or 'natural', and I steer well clear of any sort of ceremony or ritual in my work. The truth is always simple.

Healing is a matter of asking. But we also need to meet it half-way. For instance, someone suffering from deep-seated anger that has manifested itself in arthritis or cancer, needs to get to the cause of that anger if healing is to be beneficial. We can all find our own way of helping the healing by recognizing and learning from the cause of our illness. Life, after all, is about learning. It is why we are here. We need to pursue positively the adventure of being and the route we should take is the one we know to be right for our own, unique self. You are unlimited, therefore your choices in life are unlimited – it is our teachers, priests and politicians who tell us otherwise. We need to put aside all the conditioning we have had over the years and open our minds to our own, true selves. The truth about ourselves is totally indestructible and special – because it is the power that created the whole universe – it is LOVE. If you first apply this love to yourself it will follow that you will then know how best to live your life – you will not need the Ten Commandments!

The cross was a religious symbol long before it was associated with Christ. In ancient times it represented the elimination of the 'I' and this is relevant in healing – for the healer cannot heal on his own but is merely a channel for the Guv'nor's power.

When a registered osteopath came to me I had no way of knowing how healing would help him when the medical profession had been unable to do so, or, of course, of diagnosing the exact nature of the knee injury he had sustained: Jeffrey Richards D.O.(Hons), M.R.O. was in his third year studying osteopathy. Running up an escalator one day he missed his step. His left leg came down heavily and he felt an excruciating pain in the knee-cap. He limped slowly all the way home. An hour later the pain was even more severe. But as time went on – and with plenty of rest and ice treatment – the knee got a little better. Two tutors at the college examined the injury, but came up with different diagnoses. Several different types of treatment followed and the pain eased. But it never went away.

Jeff qualified and started work, but his knee became more and more painful. It was only a hundred yards from his home to the paper shop, but by the time he got there he would be in agony and would have to wait for five minutes before walking back. X-rays of his knee failed to show any damage. Ultrasound treatment was given and other osteopaths consulted. Doctors prescribed various different drugs. All to no avail.

One day a patient told Jeff how she had received relief from her pre-menstrual tension after coming for healing, and he decided to at least give it a try. Never good at relaxing, he found it difficult to unwind during the healing and it made no impression on him – although I assured him that healing had been strong. He returned to his surgery and got back to work. A friend called by and asked where he had been that morning. As Jeff recounted his visit he suddenly realized that his left knee was tingling. The sensation lasted for about half an hour, but he dismissed it as being 'all in the mind'. Later, he went upstairs to bed as usual – then had to come straight down again. For the first time in years, his knee was free of pain and he wanted to be sure he was not imagining it.

Jeff describes his second visit as 'a quite extraordinary experience. I was on a high when I left – all my senses were heightened. Even the music I played in the car on the way home seemed somehow more profound.' After a third session, Jeff reported that the problem with his knee had disappeared completely.

He says: 'I wonder now if the purpose of having the injury

was to introduce me to healing. It has helped so much in starting me off on my own spiritual journey. I have sent many of my patients to Roundstreet and most of them have benefited enormously. It has opened me up to all sorts of possibilities that I had not thought of before. It has made me more aware in my own work of including the 'mind, body and spirit' – the *whole* person – when I am treating a patient.'

A Doctor of Psychology at the Tavistock Institute came to see me on one occasion. Our conversation led to my trying to explain that we are not in fact our bodies. He had trouble grasping this. 'We need to understand the dynamics!' he insisted. I picked up the vase, containing a single pink rose, that was on the table beside me. 'But you do not have to understand the dynamics of a rose to enjoy it,' I replied.

That part of yourself which is not your body, which is sometimes called soul, spirit or individuality, is a non-material reality – an abstract. The abstract is usually assumed to be less real than the material. In fact, the opposite is true. To start with, one atom of matter is at least ninety per cent space. Your body is composed entirely of atoms, so it is at least ninety per cent not there at all! What is real is the YOU that trundles about inside the kit you call your body.

Abstracts find expression in the material but do not depend upon the material actually to exist. Let me give you an example: someone 'thought' (another abstract) the chair you are sitting on before it was actually put together. So the thought existed before the chair and will continue to exist after the material chair no longer exists as a chair. If nothing else, the thought is more real than the chair as it clearly lasts longer – it is in fact permanent.

You, too, are an abstract reality finding expression, for the short space of a lifetime, in the material of your body. You do not depend upon your body to exist, you only think you do. So it follows that you are in charge of your body; it is not in charge of you. Sometimes we need some help to put this to work and healing often provides that help, working through the part of you which is not your body. This is why the medically impossible often happens through healing.

A healer by himself heals no-one. When someone comes to me I cannot assume there will be healing for that person. But I can often sense a person's frame of mind and level of stress. Talking with them, I will usually discover what their particular need is – and this is really all part of the healing.

In the healing room the patient sits on a stool facing the window and I sit in my chair behind him. The healing power will pass through normal light clothing. I shut out everyday worries and switch on a tape of gentle music, which is relaxing for both me and the patient. And on the basis that if you want something done it is better to go to the top, I silently ask the Guv'nor for healing for the patient. If it is available I quite quickly know it – there is a strong feeling of peace and power which I feel partly in my hands.

The patient will sometimes sense the healing begin even before I have stood up, demonstrating that the power comes from beyond the healer and is simply directed through him. I have already slipped into what has been called 'the Alpha state', which is an extra quiet state of tranquillity. I then get out of my chair and place my hands very gently on the shoulders of the patient, eventually moving to the head and then slowly down the spine – the spinal cord is an extension of the brain. The healing process is very quiet and gentle. The patient may or may not feel some of what I feel – a tingling, or heat or cold. It makes my hands shake slightly and the heat or cold does not always relate to the actual temperature of my hands.

What the patient is aware of does not govern the effectiveness of healing, although the patient's awareness may assist him in the required process of change. No manipulation or massage is involved. Patients often feel healing at the location of their trouble when my hands are nowhere near it. Sometimes they can sense 'unseen hands' at work, which are not mine. When the healing power stops, I stop. Wishful thinking, either by me or the patient, plays no part. The sensation in my hands can feel stronger on one occasion than another, but this makes no difference to the healing. A recognizable change in the condition of the patient may or may not take place immediately, but in the majority of cases there is a gradual process of improvement. The patient is in the best position subsequently to assess the results, with or without medical help. He can then decide whether healing is of use to him or not and whether he wishes to have further healing sessions.

Every patient's experience is different. Joy Manvell described 'a sensation of radiation and deep relaxation'. By the time she had got home she found a renewed sense of optimism and motivation that had been lacking. She woke in the middle of the night with the feeling that someone was driving a needle into her stomach – but without the pain. Then she felt another needle in the back of her neck, and another in the base of her spine, both painless. Her back-ache, low spirits and severe migraines were all relieved. She says 'I feel that the power behind healing is a basic fact of life – a part of our world, a kind of electricity perhaps, it doesn't matter what. If we open ourselves up to it we act as a kind of transmitter – and we can then transfer this healing energy to others.'

Someone once said 'Living in the world is a matter of becoming.' You may ask yourself why we have to go through all the trials of life in the first place – but you also have to ask yourself what the alternative would be. How can we value the light without first experiencing the darkness? The fact is that everything moves – nothing stands still. The only constant in life is that everything changes all the time. So for something to exist it has to have movement. The difference between us and other life is that we alone have some choice about the direction we take. All the answers are within ourselves. We do not need to go to church, or set aside a special time to pray. Prayer is simply listening and by listening we begin to understand. To find out what is acceptable to the Guv'nor, you need only find out what is acceptable to you.

YOU are never ill, it is your body. Understanding this will help you to see that the most important and real part of you is always in good condition and able to influence your body to make the required changes from Dis-ease to Ease. You may have noticed that you do not have to be a perfect person in order to be reasonably healthy. Staying well may require some inner progress towards Ease, in order to counteract the inevitable consequences of the years. In the natural order of life the body progresses to deterioration to the point where some vital part of it ceases to work and you naturally leave the body. How comfortable the journey from the change called Life towards the change called Death may be, depends very largely upon how you choose to live that life and what attitudes you choose to adopt.

There are many healers in the world and probably as many views on healing as there are healers. I do not pretend that my views are the only ones, or indeed the only right ones. I can only speak out of my own experience, although I cannot deny that the impossible often happens in the course of my work. If a healer takes credit for any healing he must also take the blame for the failures. I prefer not to indulge in either. 'Loving Guv'nor – Thine is the Kingdom, Thine is the Power and Thine is the Glory.'

3

Why We Get Ill

You are continually building, and so externalizing in
your body, conditions most akin to the thoughts and
emotions you entertain. And not only are you so
building from within, but you are also continually
drawing from without forces of a kindred nature . . .'

Ralph Waldo Trine

Even with all the wonderful medical advances that are being
made, we do not seem to be getting any healthier! Cases of
arthritis, cancer, heart disease and depression continue to fill
our hospital beds. Doctors attempt to deal with the effects
of Dis-ease – that is, 'lack of ease' – but seldom with its
source. They acknowledge that perhaps 60 to 80 per cent of
disease is caused by stress. I believe the figure to be 100 per
cent. Whatever the source of our stress: bereavement, guilt, a
feeling of inadequacy or unresolved anger it will, given time,
find an outlet in physical or mental disease.

Research connected with the Bristol Cancer Help Centre
has shown that there is a common link between all cancer
patients – they suffer from a lack of self-esteem. This is not
to say that all those with a low opinion of themselves will get
cancer, but it is invariably true the other way round.

You have heard about the half-filled bottle of wine: we
all have the choice – to see the bottle as half-full or to
see it as half-empty. The way we think – how we interpret
events – is responsible for the way our life unfolds. There
is always trouble, always sadness if you want to look for
it – and taking the gloomy view can become a lifetime's
habit. The body takes its lead from the mind, to which it

is inextricably linked, negative thoughts inevitably drawing on and weakening our natural good health.

Illness is not an unlucky accident. We make ourselves ill by our 'lack of ease', by our wrong, conditioned thinking. When part of our body eventually ceases to function properly the surgeon gets to work. Or we become seriously depressed and the doctor gives us a bottle of pills. Medical intervention will often cure the symptoms, but our stress – our dis-ease – is still with us and will eventually reappear. Many doctors will agree that chemical drugs may not be the cure-alls once hoped for. Side-effects from drugs often outweigh any temporary benefit. And their development involves great suffering for millions of experimental animals every year.

Most people who come to see me have already been treated by orthodox medicine which for one reason or another has not proved successful. I see many patients who are suffering from cancer or depression, often at an advanced stage. It may be the first time in years, perhaps ever, that the patient has had the opportunity to speak and hear about the reality of his spiritual being – about what he *is* rather than what he merely *does*. I remind my patients that *we* are in charge of our mind and body and can, therefore, *choose* to be well. From time to time though, everyone needs a little help. And that help is available in the form of healing.

We all fall into habits of attitude or reaction and it can take time to change a way of thinking or behaving that we have always assumed to be right, not recognizing the damage it has been causing. Yet *the guidance needed to achieve ease is already inside you.* It has been called conscience, goodness or love. Even the most wicked man loves something, if only himself. No man has less love within him than any other – but it is a matter of how much we will allow that spark within to function. The love within us is not rationed. A person's attitude to their illness will make all the difference to the quality of their life – and a positive attitude can actually bring about a physical change for the better.

Two charming ladies in their eighties came one day for healing. They walked through the door carefully, hanging on to each other and laughing helplessly. It turned out that they both had great difficulty in walking unaided. One of the ladies tended to veer off to the left instead of keeping in a straight line and the other would sometimes find herself toppling backwards. To solve the problem they had hit on the solution of going everywhere together, each keeping the other upright and moving in the right direction! Rather than give up in despair, they had chosen to see the humour of the situation, hence the giggles and great sense of fun. It takes courage to laugh at ourselves, but these two friends had found that courage. With their navigation greatly improved, they were able to do their own shopping which had been impossible before. Their approach to life was such a tonic, I am not sure who healed whom that day!

To whatever extent you think little of yourself, you are being rather rude to the Guv'nor! It was He who created you unique, warts and all, in the first place. By denying your own uniqueness and importance, you are in effect saying that He does not know what He is doing, or that He is only half in charge. If you do not think of yourself as totally special, it is time you started, because that is what you are! It is of course nothing to do with being big-headed – there is a fundamental difference between what you *do* and what you actually *are*.

I always explain the philosophy behind the healing – that we existed before we joined up with our body at birth, and will exist after we leave the 'kit' behind. And in the meantime, to get well and stay that way, we need to be a little kinder to ourselves. This may perhaps be a new and difficult line of thought for someone trained on 'It is better to give than to receive', but as with everything else, we need to practise new skills.

I have found that it is what healing implies that often has the most profound effect. The patient comes to understand that this is a direct contact with what is beyond our present existence and experience – evidence of the power of love that is eternal. Healing can restore not only health, but also hope.

Did you know that you are invisible? I once had a

patient who came to me suffering with an acute lack of self-confidence – she was extremely shy and retiring and this had almost ruined her life. What I told her took her very much by surprise: 'If you understand that you and your body are two different things then it follows that no-one can see you – they can only see your body. If you know this, what reason do you have for being so shy? Why not test it out – run up the street with no clothes on! People will either be shocked or amused, but they will certainly not be looking at YOU – just the kit you were born with.' My patient had a good laugh at this – and of course laughter itself is a great healer!

Valuing ourselves and our individual point of view is important if we are to lead stress-free, healthy lives. For instance, we all at one time or another experience unpleasantness or unkindness from others. If we can ignore this – make nothing of it – it ceases to be a reality. It is only real, only a problem, if we make it so. By becoming involved with the other person's behaviour we are simply adding to their burden of anger or jealousy, whatever it is, by making it actual fact. No-one gains by it. Let it go. Agree if necessary, even if you know them to be wrong, because in this way their spite has nowhere else to go.

Keep your own counsel. It is part of the kindness you owe to yourself. I always tell my patients: *you* are totally special. If someone else does not recognize this, it is their problem not yours, unless you choose to make it so. This attitude may, of course, take some time to cultivate. But it is worth the effort. The following example clearly illustrates the point.

A woman in her forties came to me, struggling painfully on two sticks. A friend had to help her into the room. For many years she had been semi-paralysed from the waist down. She told me that doctors had carried out every conceivable medical test. They had told her they could discover nothing physically wrong. Although she came to me on a number of occasions, healing did not happen. During our various conversations, I began to find out more about my patient. Her widowed mother had depended on her to act as a nurse until the day she died – all the time treating my patient like a child, sending her to bed early every evening and allowing her no freedom to live her own life. When my patient asked her mother's permission to marry she gave it, but on one condition: that the couple came to live with her after the wedding. This they did, but the mother's tyrannical behaviour was soon directed towards her son-in-law as well.

By the time my patient came to me she had a teenage son and her mother had died. But in the mother's will the house had been left jointly to her daughter and her own sister, so my patient's aunt had come to live with them. The hatred for her mother was consequently transferred to her aunt.

One day my patient went on holiday to Spain with her husband and son, leaving her aunt at home. She told me that the moment she stepped out of the plane at Malaga the paralysis disappeared. This continued until she arrived back at Gatwick, when the condition suddenly reappeared. I talked about this to my patient and suggested that she was bringing the paralysis on herself, although unwittingly. She was not impressed with this idea. I also one day suggested that, on her way home, she should buy a lovely bunch of flowers for her aunt. The look on my patient's face said it all. 'Oh no, I couldn't do that. She will probably throw them back at me' was her immediate reaction. I said that if her aunt did not accept the flowers it really did not matter – just try it and see how things go. Why not make a start at bringing some happiness into a home you share with another? But she would not change her mind. Her paralysis was still troubling her when I last saw her and she has now stopped coming. This, to my mind, is a classic case of dis-ease: lack of ease from all the anger she had stored up, finding expression in the body.

There are, unfortunately, some people who enjoy being ill, even if this is unconscious on their part. A woman of about sixty came to Roundstreet with a long list of ailments. When she came in to see me she was wearing a surgical collar, which she removed when she sat down. I asked her what was wrong with her neck. 'Oh,' she said, 'there is nothing actually wrong with my neck, but you never know – I might have a car accident!' She was very keen to talk. For once I had to do most of the listening! One of the things concerning her was that she had no friends. It turned out that she had had a very unhappy life. The problem was obviously connected with her father, but I never found out what exactly had been wrong. She discovered, after her marriage, that her husband was a homosexual. This of course did nothing for her self-esteem. They eventually split up. In spite of all her – I believe largely imagined – ills, I could tell that she was a very thoughtful and kindly person. One day I put it to her: 'Has it ever crossed your mind that you may actually enjoy being ill?'

She brightened up at once. 'Do you know,' she said, 'that's exactly what my doctor said to me.' She then immediately changed the subject. It was obviously something she did not want to look at. It seemed to me that my patient's need to talk, always at great length, was a result of the loneliness and unhappiness she felt. But this meant that her problem was self-perpetuating, her ceaseless chatter driving away the friends she so much wanted to make. This, perhaps, was why she relied on being ill as a way of bringing to herself the attention and comfort she needed.

A Sussex psychiatrist, Doctor Graham Shepherd, has conducted a study of attitudes to therapy. His findings are encouraging. He believes people are now more open to the idea that the body is affected, whether positively or negatively, by the mind. Young men, he says, are not afraid to admit that they cry – the natural releasing of emotion that their fathers and grandfathers would probably have considered a weakness. More people are keen to attend relaxation classes as they begin to understand that right thinking can actually affect the chemical balance of their bodies. It is a proven fact, he says, that breast cancer patients can relapse if under stress and the death of a partner can bring on cancer or a stroke.

Stress – even if we do not recognize it – affects us all, including children. Richard was suffering with a continuous round of crippling migraines at the age of ten. Painkillers did not help and his school work was affected. After healing, the migraines lessened and then eventually vanished altogether for a year. Now, with an occasional 'top-up', Richard can keep them well under control.

It often happens that healing brings people to a clearer understanding of the real cause of their dis-ease. When they recognize the burden they are dragging along with them they can begin to off-load it, and this is how they begin to get better. Whatever the physical complaint – arthritis for instance, asthma or migraines – whenever the patient becomes angry, disturbed or upset the symptoms will re-occur. The link between stress and disease is undisputable.

People sometimes comment that it is all very well telling them to change their way of thinking, but old habits die hard. I know this can be true, but in fact being ill is much more difficult than being well. So it should become progressively easier as you strive to change those old habits. When you begin to connect the improvements you feel in your body with the discarding of your negative attitudes, life will begin to look much more hopeful.

A woman in her seventies was still suffering from terrible anger at the way she had been treated at her boarding school before the age of eighteen. I tried to make her see the senselessness of continuing to bear the weight of these memories; that she should begin closing the door on this part of her past. The only person she could hurt, by harbouring this bitterness, was herself (the teachers concerned having long since departed this world). But she somehow felt she could not let go of it.

I tell people they should be glad of their anger. If you have never become really angry about something, you have also never had the opportunity to think about a preferable alternative. We are all moving on and changing continuously. We need to learn the lesson our anger is teaching us and then leave the anger behind when it is no longer of use to us. By taking it with us, we not only damage ourselves but also affect those around us. We all sense each other's unhappiness. Without knowing what is troubling a person, we detect the ambiance of that trouble when we meet them. Those who are sought out by others are the people 'at ease' with themselves. Because that ease, like laughter, is infectious!

It does happen sometimes that a patient who comes to see me is so unhappy, he or she is contemplating suicide. One man I spoke to could no longer find a reason to continue with his life. He was in utter despair. I asked him to think about what would happen if, on arriving at the gates of Heaven, St Peter said 'Get lost! You're not due here for another twenty-five years!' My patient's mood was too black for him to even raise a smile at this. But it made him think. In time, he found his outlook on life did improve.

I have always believed that stress accounts for not just some but, in one way or another, all diseases. Emotions have a direct effect upon the body. Anger causes muscle tension: witness the clenched fist of an angry man. If you just *think* about sucking a lemon your mouth will react with saliva – a good example of how thought affects us physically. And there are other, more subtle influences at work in our lives. Some ideas, taken for granted from an early age and even assumed to be good, can be very harmful. Most people would automatically agree with the statement 'It is better to give than to receive.' But this is not right. Giving and receiving are exactly the same thing. If you have ever loved anyone you will know this to be true. Perhaps whoever invented 'It is better to give' had a collection plate in his hand at the time! The implication of it is that one is somehow lessened by receiving.

One of the tapes I use in my healing sessions starts with the sound of the sea. I usually tell patients about the tape they are going to hear before I start, but on one occasion I forgot. My patient, an elderly woman suffering with arthritis, was poised on the stool in the healing room. However, the minute the sound of waves on the shore reached her ears she rushed from the room, explaining that she had to find the loo. On her return I remarked that she had obviously been potty-trained to the sound of a tap! She said that this was quite true, and that it had been a problem for her all her life. I explained that the message she was receiving – that she had to make a run for it every time she heard the sound of water

– had first to go through her ears and mind. But her ears and mind belonged to *her* – *she* was in control. And she could decide to take no notice of the message if that was what she wanted. She told me later that she had quickly been able to stop the habit, even though she had lived with it for seventy years. Her arthritis also got better!

Stress (or dis-ease) will always prevent the body functioning naturally and will interfere with its enormous capacity to heal itself, given the right help or stimulation. All the wonderful techniques employed by doctors actually do no more than this. Unfortunately medical intervention is often more of an imposition upon the body – witness the sometimes terrible side-effects of modern drugs. My view of healing is that taking the design (the human being) back to the designer for repair is probably the most effective method of getting it fixed. All the best things happen in peace and quiet.

Turmoil and disharmony are not conducive to beneficial change. It is up to us how much tranquillity exists within us. For instance, there is nothing compulsory about being miserable when it is raining!

The opposite of dis-ease is *ease*. And cultivating our inner tranquillity is the beginning of healing, as my patient, Wendy Galleymore, found. At thirty-seven, Wendy was abruptly struck down by a crippling disease. She woke up with terrible pain in her neck and arms. X-rays showed that she was suffering with osteo-arthritis and her doctor said it was unlikely she would be able to work again. 'Put it down to your age' was the only explanation she received. All the nerve endings in her arm were inflamed and she faced the prospect of wearing a surgical collar and undergoing extensive physiotherapy. She could not turn her head without turning her whole body. With a marriage that was breaking up and two children to look after, she was in despair. She was not convinced healing would help, but this is how she described her experience:

When someone in great pain is given relief, it is not just the physical body that is healed. Strength, too, comes from the knowledge that the healing power is available to us. This strength helped me look at the stress that had made me ill in the first place.

I have always been a tense, anxious person and when I first sat on that stool I felt more nervous than ever. Then Phil put on some music and I began to relax. Suddenly I felt what I can only describe as a rectangle of heat in my back – and this was before he had touched me. It was like a mild electric shock. I was embarrassed to find myself crying, but I could not help it. I just felt an overwhelming sense of peace sitting there. When I came out I went back to the waiting room as my friend's mother was going in for healing after me. For some time I had been having sleepless nights, no position being comfortable for long because of the pain. However, after the healing I fell fast asleep. My friend, sitting with me, was concerned that my head was bent over, resting on my arm. She thought I might wake up in agony, as would previously have been the case. But Phil told her not to worry, that I would be alright – and I was. From then on the pain gradually disappeared and, after one more visit, it has never returned.

I continue to keep an open mind about spiritual matters. I was impressed when a medium was able to give an accurate analysis of my character and difficulties. Having done no more than ask my name, she immediately told me I would have to toughen up a bit. She said that there was someone in my life making me unhappy, but if I stood up to him I would be alright. 'You must stop letting people walk all over you.' She was absolutely right. I have always been the sort of person who did just that, unable ever to say No. She was describing not only how I was behaving, but also the situation between my husband and myself at the time.

I am now free of pain and leading a normal life. The sense of peace and well-being I felt during healing was so intense, I remember thinking at the time that, even if the pain did not go, it would not matter. For the first time in my life I was at one with myself. Healing saved my life.

Sometimes we find it hard to believe what seems to be impossible – we think we can't change and get well. Or perhaps, because we fear the changes it will bring to our lives, we do not even *want* to get well. This reminds me of the caterpillar who looked up one day from the leaf he was munching and saw a beautiful butterfly go flying by. 'Mm,' he said to himself, you'd never get me up in one of those things!'

4

Beyond Medical Experience

Flee from the crowd and dwell in truthfulness
Suffice you with your gifts, though they be small
To hoard brings hate, to climb brings giddiness
The crowd has envy, and success blinds all
Desire no more than to your lot may fall
Work well yourself, to counsel others clear
And truth shall make you free, there is no fear!

Chaucer

From my experience of healing I have found that absolutely nothing is impossible. Beneficial changes in mind or body do not depend on the state of knowledge of the medical establishment at any given time. After all, man's collective wisdom is just a fraction of all there is yet to know. The telephone was possible a million years ago because the materials of which it is made have always been with us. The only thing missing, until recently, was man's understanding of how to put it together. Healing is proof of an intelligence greater than we can comprehend. Some of the beneficial changes my patients have experienced both during and after healing would, in orthodox medicine, have needed an anaesthetic. Yet the patient feels no pain, even if he or she is aware that something is happening.

Twelve-year-old Tamsin Atley was not very enthusiastic at the idea of coming for healing. Born with a dislocated hip after a breach birth, she had her leg in a splint for three months as a baby. This seemed to put matters right, but from the age of seven and for the next five years she was in such pain she could at times hardly walk or even stand. She had seen several doctors during this time, and as there was still no sign of any improvement, she did not expect that healing could help.

When Tamsin first complained of pains in her right heel her parents took her to a consultant who diagnosed Severs Disease (where the bone and muscle grow at different rates). As time went on the pain gradually got worse. Having a fighting spirit, Tamsin still tried to join in with games at school, but this soon became impossible. She began to suffer intense throbbing pain and heat in her foot and her General Practitioner prescribed a strong drug for ten days which gave temporary relief, but the pain returned soon afterwards. A different consultant X-rayed her foot and made the same diagnosis. He told her that the pain would disappear within four months, but it steadily increased and she found she could walk only short distances. Physiotherapy did not bring any improvement either.

The original consultant took another X-ray and this time decided the problem was *not* Severs Disease. Tamsin's leg was put in plaster which brought only temporary relief, and four weeks later the plaster was removed and a cortisone injection given. After this the pain got worse and worse, with swelling and throbbing all the time. A bone scan and blood test showed nothing more than heat in the right ankle. Tamsin began taking painkillers and a muscle relaxant but could hardly walk by this time or concentrate at school. The pain got so bad that it hurt just to touch the skin.

A doctor at Great Ormond Street Hospital in London said that the pain would ease in time, but this did not prove to be the case and Tamsin was taken to see yet another consultant. Her mother tried aromatherapy, but the pain got no better.

When the Atley's G.P. suggested another referral, they decided instead to give healing a try. After a month of weekly healing sessions, Tamsin was able to stop taking the muscle relaxant pills. A few months later she stopped taking painkillers and was able to walk long distances without any pain.

Tamsin soon overcame her initial doubts and was able to relax and talk easily. She reports feeling calm and sleepy after the first visit, after which there was some easement of the pain. A slight relapse followed. But after subsequent visits her foot slowly but surely healed. She is now making up for lost time – she rides, walks the dog, gardens and plays tennis. Her parents have great difficulty slowing her down, and still cannot get used to the sight of their daughter running up and down the stairs!

None of the causes of any physical ailment is anywhere in the body. It is a waste of time to give a corpse an aspirin – there is no-one there. Everything that happens to the body is because you are in it. This is not a matter of fault or blame. It is merely a reflection of the fact that living in the world is so stressful that in the end it kills us all. The stress we all experience often manifests itself in migraines, and many people seek healing for this condition when orthodox medicine has been unable to help.

Frederick Cridland, a semi-retired chiropodist in his late seventies, had suffered with severe migraine headaches since childhood. Although the severity of the headaches became less as he got older, over more recent years the migraines had been causing blind spots. His specialist told him that, as a result of all the headaches and pain of the past, the optic nerve had been damaged and that nothing could be done about it. The 'half-blindness' eased for a while after Freddie cut down his workload, but it eventually came back. He found he could suddenly only see half a person's face. On one occasion, because he could not see where he was going, he hit the kerb while driving and found himself changing a burst tyre in the pouring rain.

Freddie also suffered with Raynaud's Syndrome, a condition where the fingers or toes lose all sensation and turn white. The nerve becomes frozen and shuts down, in turn shutting off all the blood vessels and occasionally leading to gangrene.

After the first healing session, Freddie found that his fingers did not go white and lifeless, as they would normally have done, while he was clearing snow on a bitterly cold day. A few days later he had the beginnings of half-blindness at work. But after five minutes the condition had resolved itself. After a second visit for healing, Freddie experienced no more bad headaches or blindness. The Raynaud's Syndrome also cleared, and he reported feeling generally better, despite having some personal problems at the time.

For a woman in her early forties who had suffered for two years with a devastating skin complaint, recovery was both rapid and dramatic. The condition flared up every three months or so and lasted for two weeks at a time. It would start with an itchy rash on her arms and wrists and then spread to her face, turning into little bumps under the skin. Her skin would become progressively hotter and redder 'like very bad sunburn – if I held my hand near my face I could feel the heat. Just as though it was on fire.' Eventually her skin would dry out and crack and her eyes swelled up until they were reduced to weeping slits. Doctors did not know what it was, and although they prescribed cortisone creams and injections, nothing worked. Allergy testing also drew a blank.

The day following her first visit for healing, my patient reports feeling 'completely renewed and exhilarated. I felt I could have done anything – as though I had taken some marvellous drug!' After one more visit her skin complaint vanished completely and has not come back since.

Medicine today is based almost entirely on science, and some doctors are still unwilling to consider cures that cannot be measured scientifically. But the mood in the medical profession is gradually changing: in its recent publication *Complementary Medicine – New Approaches to Good Practice*, the British Medical Association's Board of Science and Education advocate closer collaboration between the medical profession and practitioners of non-conventional medicine for clinical research.

I was delighted, early on in my practice, to meet a medical doctor who had an open mind about the possibilities of healing. Dr Priscilla Noble-Mathews came to see me after a close friend of hers was relieved of her migraines following two sessions of healing. She was impressed by what she had heard, and we had several long talks about healing and my views on it. Dr Noble-Mathews believed that healing could be complementary to orthodox medicine, which she felt was too quick to prescribe drugs rather than consider a patient's underlying stress.

I have always hoped for closer co-operation between healers and the medical profession, and was very pleased when Dr Noble-Mathews agreed to undertake some joint research with me. With the prior agreement of patients who were willing to take part, the doctor would make an initial examination, then check the patient's progress, after visits for healing, by scientific medical methods. When patients were referred to me by Priscilla, she did not tell me anything about them except their name. She left me to find out their problems. I felt that if healing could be proved to the medical profession, this would help to advance scientific knowledge and be of benefit to all.

Our joint research project was approved by The Koestler Foundation, which was set up to encourage research into unorthodox methods of treating disease. Dr Richard Tonkin, a Fellow of the Royal College of Physicians, was on its panel of advisors. He came down to advise Priscilla and me on the setting up of the project, which was described in the Foundation's brochure as 'a longitudinal study of the effects of hand-healing'.

An office and small surgery were prepared and furnished in the coach-house for use by Dr Noble-Mathews. Here she saw her private patients and, where she thought it appropriate, advised them to come to me.

Although it was supported by The Koestler Foundation, the Roundstreet Project did not attract the attention of any benefactor for much-needed funds. Sue's Pools win could in no way have covered the costs of the medical research which it was planned to set up. Then, regretfully, Dr Noble-Mathews moved away to another practice outside the area. But I did not give up hope that the kind of collaboration we had started would one day be continued.

Increasingly, orthodox medical practitioners are becoming

interested in the work of genuine healers, and some seek healing themselves. David Soltau FRCS, FRCOG, a surgeon living in Gloucestershire, has written the following personal account:

I was brought up in an orthodox medical household, as my father and grandfather were both doctors. In the 1930s my father's cousin, a surgeon on the staff of a famous London hospital, used to stay with us in the country for occasional weekends. As an impressionable teenager I listened with interest to medical talk between him and my father. Sometimes I heard the eminent surgeon speak with contempt of the iniquities of 'faith healers', who seemed to him to be mere charlatans, and I came to realize that the healing miracles in the Bible no longer seemed relevant with the advent of 'modern' medicine and surgery.

In due course I qualified in medicine myself, and after Army service in the Far East I spent several years in a variety of hospitals training as a specialist in a branch of surgery, eventually becoming a hospital consultant. This was a busy and demanding post, and I thought no more of healing or healers, though I became aware that occasionally patients under my care had also been treated by a healer. When this was discussed at a hospital committee meeting I said that I could see no harm in this practice provided it did not replace orthodox medical or surgical treatment. This, of course, was after 1977, the year when the General Medical Council rescinded its ban on doctors associating with 'unqualified practitioners' such as healers or osteopaths.

One day, after I had retired from hospital work, I happened to watch the final few minutes of a TV programme on healing, and this aroused my interest in the subject. In a bookshop the next day I came across Phil Edwardes' remarkable book *Healing for You*. I bought it, and read it from cover to cover with the greatest interest. The book was a revelation! Here were detailed accounts of patients with intractable medical and surgical problems who had reached the end of the road with orthodox medical treatment, but were still plagued with discomfort, pain and disability. Yet after healing sessions with Phil Edwardes (not 'faith-healing', as no faith was required) they obtained great benefit; in some cases so marked as to be really miraculous. The book was modestly written, the healer himself claiming no credit or medical knowledge, but ascribing the healing process to God, or the 'Guv'nor'. My interest was stimulated, and I discussed the question of healing with an Anglican clergyman who had a considerable local reputation as a healer. He told me of some amazing cases from his own experience, which increased my interest so that I decided to investigate further.

For several years I had suffered from a mild form of arthritis which caused backache and stiffness of the spine, and for which I took analgesic and anti-inflammatory tablets from time to time. This condition was associated with painful attacks of eye inflammation (iritis or uveitis), which necessitated the use of steroid eye-drops for a few weeks or so. These attacks occurred every year or two and were inconvenient though not incapacitating. However, in the two years preceding my retirement they had become more frequent. Now the thought struck me! Why not try healing?

A visit to Phil Edwardes appealed to me more than the idea of attending a crowded healing service in a church, but I remained apprehensive about the plan, although I knew that healing could not aggravate my condition. Accordingly, I wrote to Phil and had an encouraging reply. There was nothing to lose, so I made an appointment.

An interesting talk took place and I was pleased to find that Phil believed in the importance of co-operation of healing with orthodox medicine. It was not necessary to abandon the latter if one received healing. At this first session I experienced a slight feeling of warmth and a mild tingling sensation. but nothing else. However, Phil assured me that healing had been present, which was a relief.

Two days later my left eye appeared red, but not painful. This was not a true attack of iritis and the condition was transitory, so no eye-drops were needed. I attended for further healing sessions with marked benefit, and apart from one very mild episode of iritis I have had no further trouble and have been free from attacks for the past four years.

My spine, also, has shown a marked improvement. I still have mild backache from time to time, but nothing like the pain and stiffness I suffered in the past. However, as a small measure of 'self-help' I take generous doses of vitamins A and D in the form of halibut-liver oil capsules, beneficial in certain types of arthritis as well as in eye problems.

A cataract in my right eye became troublesome, a sequel to the steroid eye-drops used in the past as well as advancing age. To my great relief, a most successful operation was performed, with a lens implant that resulted in perfect vision. A similar operation was performed on the left eye a year later, again with an excellent result and no complications.

In the meantime my wife had been a sufferer from migraines for many years, her headaches being so bad at times that she had to have a day in bed. Phil Edwardes kindly treated her as well, with enormous improvement. Now the worst that happens is an occasional slight headache, which responds quickly to mild analgesics.

I have enjoyed many fascinating discussions on healing with Phil, and much appreciate his sensible, down-to-earth approach. I realize that there are many other avenues of healing and that some may prefer a church service with laying-on of hands by the clergy. Although a regular church-goer myself, I must admit that I find the atmosphere of healing services somewhat over-emotional, and I greatly prefer the simple, personal approach to that of a large assembly. I am also wary of those healers who decry all orthodox medical treatment, and strongly support the opinion that a joint approach of healing and medicine has the most to offer.

Thankfully mutual respect and co-operation between medical practitioners and healers is becoming more common. But there are still many who prefer to speak of 'spontaneous remission', 'incorrect medical diagnosis' or even 'psychosomatic' when healing cannot be explained in scientific terms. If a drug company finds that a particular drug has even a modest success rate, millions of pounds are poured into funding promotion and further research. That healing does not attract similar financial resources is perhaps due to the fact that its very nature means that there are no huge financial gains to be made. And yet thousands of patients have received lasting benefit from it, without any side-effects of the kind associated with powerful drugs.

Nineteen-year-old Sara Crow was keen to try an alternative treatment to the painkillers and anti-inflammatory tablets that were being prescribed for her painful arthritic condition, ankylosing spondylitis.

From her first visit for healing there was a dramatic improvement in Sara's condition. The pain in her spine was so much reduced that she was able to cut down the number of pills she was taking. Soon she had given them up completely. She also found it helpful to talk over the worries she had at the time with someone outside her circle of family and friends.

At first, Sara came for healing every three weeks, then every few months, depending on how she felt. She saw her specialist only once more and was told she looked better and that her back was straighter. She had always been reluctant to take the drugs prescribed for her and was delighted when she found she no longer needed them. I encouraged her to take up swimming and she has found that gentle exercise of this sort helps with the steady improvement in her spine.

There is only one 'constant' in life, and that is that everything changes all the time. Even the apparently inert rock is neither solid nor still. Science explains that there is no such thing as a solid, that all matter is energy – the same energy finding expression in different ways. This is very close to the age-old assertion that God is all or that it is all 'The One'. The rock has little choice about the changes that occur within it, but we *do* have choice about the changes that occur within the matter or energy that makes up our bodies. Far more choice in fact than is currently assumed by modern medicine. Science clings to the idea that if something cannot be measured on the laboratory bench it does not exist. This makes it difficult to consider the reality of what is non-material. Does the scientist ignore the fact that he loves his wife because he cannot measure that love?

Many people seek healing as a last resort – when conventional treatment has perhaps already been abandoned. This was the case for a young female medical practitioner who, desperate to start a family but unable to achieve a successful pregnancy, had gone through every possible medical test and form of treatment.

When ovulation predictor tests indicated that she was not ovulating for three months in succession, she went to see her own G.P. He wasn't too worried and advised her to return if she still wasn't pregnant after a further nine months. When she did return, he referred her to a specialist, having verified that her husband's sperm count was normal.

From the blood test results, polycystic ovarian disease was diagnosed. At first, the patient's anxiety was allayed by the doctor when he told her that eighty per cent of women respond to drug treatment. But after three months, further tests showed she was not responding well enough to the drug and the prescription was changed. Some months later the treatment was changed again, and a new drug had to be injected on alternate days. My patient had to collect all her urine and send a sample to the laboratory every other day for testing so that the drug dose could be precisely gauged. But the months passed, bringing only disappointment. One night, my patient found herself arriving at the Savoy Hotel in London in her ball gown, clutching a large canister three-quarters full of urine – disguised only by a carrier bag. She found it difficult to make a graceful entrance with a large volume of liquid sloshing audibly, and was relieved that the cloakroom attendant was too busy to notice what she had given her!

When a pregnancy test proved positive my patient and her husband felt that at last their troubles were over. But at nine weeks she miscarried and the treatment regime had to start all over again.

When urine tests showed a risk of drug overdose, the treatment was halted, and replaced by ultra-sound scans. Getting time off work to attend for the scans was difficult and added to the stress of the situation.

After three years of raised hopes and disappointments, despair was beginning to creep in. Treatment finally came to a stop a few months later when it became obvious that my patient was one of the unlucky twenty per cent who did not respond.

It was at this point that she decided to give healing a try. She was disappointed, on her visit, that she felt no sensation of any sort, but I was able to assure her that I had felt a lot of healing during the session. She reported afterwards that, driving along a country lane the following day and thinking of nothing in particular, she suddenly felt different – full of energy and enthusiasm. 'It occurred as suddenly as if a light switch had been turned on – and the effect was very similar.'

A repeat of the original tests, as well as new investigations, were started at the Hammersmith Hospital the same day, and a week later my patient came for her second session of healing. The following month a scan at the hospital showed that the cysts, which had been clearly present on the ovaries on a previous scan, had now vanished. She continued to come for healing, as well as undergoing a battery of tests at the Hammersmith Hospital – although no treatment – for the next three months. Blood tests which had previously been abnormal now came back 100 per cent normal.

A few weeks later a pregnancy test showed positive. My patient later wrote: 'We could not believe our luck, but the evidence is here and beaming at me from his baby bouncer as I write this! I subsequently learnt from Professor Winston at the Hammersmith Hospital that polycystic ovarian disease can occasionally disappear of its own accord. However, I did not know that until eighteen months later. I am certain that my recovery was due to the healing I received. I had not had any conventional treatment for several months and it had been abandoned as it was not achieving its desired result. The altered state that I described the day after my first healing session was extraordinarily powerful, almost intoxicating. The transformation was quite unprovoked by me and so dramatic that it actually felt as though a miracle had occurred at that moment. This would appear to be borne out by the various medical tests that followed. I am in no doubt that the healing was responsible for our long-desired bouncing baby miracle.'

Medical science, with all its skills, continues to deal almost exclusively with the body. It is therefore only dealing with effects. The human body is a marvel of design at work. It is too complex and beautiful to be an unguided accident or a machine. We own, and to some extent consciously control, our bodies – and to some extent we unconsciously control them. Sometimes we do not do this very well and describe ourselves as being affected by some ailment or dis-ease. Medical science can and often does help, but still only deals with the physical. Healing deals with the whole person and therefore the causes of the ailment are included in the treatment. This can never happen, though, against the free-will of the patient. Healing cannot be imposed – it is merely offered. This is because the source of healing is Love and Love itself never insists.

I have no text book to work by. Every healer works in the way that seems best to him. And because every patient is different, there can be no set rules.

Another 'miracle baby' is Max. His mother, Sandra Rowley,

had been suffering from endometriosis, a disease that causes infertility in nine out of ten cases. Her doctor had even stopped prescribing the contraceptive pill, as there no longer seemed any point in taking it. And Sandra had to try and come to terms with the fact that she would never have a family of her own.

In endometriosis the cells lining the womb begin to grow outside the womb, affecting the fallopian tubes. Sandra had been to hospital for two operations for cysts and was in pain most of the time. The only treatment doctors could offer was a course of male hormones. This stops the periods and can have undesirable side-effects like deepening of the voice and facial hair! Sandra gave up the treatment when her skin erupted in boils. Just before this she began having severe stomach cramps again. Healing had been helpful in alleviating a period of stress two years before, and she decided to give it another try.

Two months later Sandra began having stomach pains again. As she was due to have another hospital check-up the following month, this was brought forward. She had begun to bleed and assumed that the endometriosis had flared up again with another cyst. The hospital kept her in overnight. The next morning they announced that she was pregnant. Tests to check the position and progress of the baby also showed that there was no sign at all of the endometriosis.

When a patient arrives for a healing session, we first sit and talk so that I may discover how the patient feels and what the ailment may be – where it hurts, and when. I make notes, but not a medical record of any sort, just to record the 'score' at the time of the first visit, so that we may later refer to it to see how things may have changed. I also make sure that the patient is not substituting healing for his medical attention, as both can help when both are being applied, as they did for Captain Edward Graham. He had cataracts in both eyes, as well as a haemorrhage behind the left eye. The haemorrhage could not be removed by surgery and, as it was of long standing, was unlikely to disappear. Doctors had therefore decided to remove the cataract from the right eye in due course and to leave the left eye alone. Captain Graham knew of friends who had consulted healers, and it seemed worthwhile to see if anything could be done about the haemorrhage in the left eye before the removal of the cataract in the right eye.

He was relieved when I assured him that no conventional religious faith was necessary in healing. Captain Graham describes himself as the strictly no-nonsense type, but he was struck by the sensation of extreme well-being during healing. After several sessions the sight of the left eye steadily improved, to the surprise of the eye specialist. The haemorrhage is still in evidence, but far less of an inconvenience. The removal of the cataract from the right eye was a success and, with the improved left eye, his eyesight is much better than could have been anticipated.

If you tried running through a door without opening it and you broke your neck, the coroner might say the reason for your neck being broken is that your head hit the door, and the marks on your face prove it. He would be quite wrong. The reason for your broken neck would be that you didn't think to open the door. So the real cause would not be a physical cause. Medical science mostly treats physical results, and thank God for the doctors! Healing treats the *causes* and therefore also the results.

When she was fourteen, Nicola Grellis slipped and fell against a bolt on her horse-box, injuring the base of her spine. The excrutiating pain she felt at the time was to continue, on and off, for many years to come. Various falls from ponies aggravated the condition. In addition to the pain in her back, the injury had travelled up her spine to her neck and shoulders, causing severe headaches, and she often had shooting pains in her right leg. None of the osteopaths or doctors she subsequently visited had been able to do much to alleviate the problem.

Nicola's life-style (she is a game farmer and also keeps horses and several large dogs) means that she is constantly on the move, often lifting and carrying heavy weights. Eighteen years after the original accident, she was in such pain she did not know where to turn for help. 'I had this blinding headache the whole time. I just didn't know what to do.' She lives only a couple of miles away from Roundstreet House, and a friend advised her to book an appointment. She admits that she was terribly sceptical and came along with the attitude that healing could not possibly work. She arrived in a very bad state: 'The headache was so bad I was seeing stars and I had this shooting pain in my leg. I was taking very strong painkillers at the time, prescribed by the doctor. I was also under a great deal of stress. My father was dying, and I'm sure this was contributing to how ill I felt. In the healing room Phil told me to clear my mind, so I concentrated on the bowl of roses on the window sill in front of me. He put on some very soothing classical music, which I loved, so I found it quite easy to relax. He put his hands first on my shoulders, then on my head. I had the sensation of everything just dropping away – the pain, tension, everything – all falling away under his hands. There was a tingling coming from his hands too. I remember feeling very, very cold afterwards. As soon as I got home I fell into a dead sleep for two hours.'

Nicola later telephoned and left a message with the secretary – to let me know that the headache and pain had completely vanished as she walked out of the healing room!

Some months later Nicola fell and slipped a disc. After a week she went to see a physiotherapist, then after a further week, came to see me. Nicola says she again did not expect much from healing, but left with a lot of the pain having 'fallen away'.

'I sat on the stool and as I relaxed I could almost feel myself falling off – but I was too relaxed to do anything about it. I can remember thinking or hoping that if I did fall, Phil would catch me. Afterwards, as I had done the first time, I felt very cold and once again I slept for several hours when I got home. For 24 hours afterwards there was very little pain, but as I then did move about more, the discomfort returned. Having said that, I did not feel that it was necessary to return for healing, as the pain was certainly not so acute as it had been before and, five weeks on, I am well on the mend. I found my physio willing to listen with interest to my experience. Another time I would make sure I went for healing straight away, instead of hoping to get better on my own.

When healing is effective, some people recover very quickly. Much more often it is a process of beneficial change happening gradually and requiring a number of sessions. When it is gradual it can also be a matter of 'two steps forward and one back'. If you begin to get better it means you *can* get better, although it may require some perseverance on your part. Here at Roundstreet there are no rules about how often a patient comes for healing. As with medical treatment, you will know sooner or later how you feel, and it is something that you will know better than anyone else. So it is my patients who decide how often they attend – not me!

Audrey had already undergone an operation on her right ear before she came to see me. Doctors had performed microsurgery, taking a piece of vein tissue from her foot and grafting it onto the hammer bone. She had become deaf in her left ear some years before and wore a hearing aid. Before the operation her hearing was very 'muzzy' and she was unable to distinguish words clearly, and although afterwards there was some improvement, she found that she was turning up the volume on her hearing aid more and more as time went on.

In Audrey's case, beneficial change seemed to bring about a temporary turn for the worse. She said that she felt as though she had contracted a bad case of flu after the healing session – aching in every bone and joint. Wherever she had had an injury or problem in the past, the discomfort was particularly noticeable – with a terrible ache in her right ear.

The morning after her first visit, Audrey's husband spoke to her and she answered without difficulty. They were both astonished to realize that she could clearly hear every word

– and she had not yet put in her hearing aid. This would have been impossible before.

She has been back three times, and her hearing is better now than it had been with the hearing aid. The first time she came, she fell asleep and I had to wake her up. Another time she found herself in tears. She tells me she always goes back home with a cold! Audrey did not expect an instant miracle and finds that her hearing can again become muzzy at times. But healing always helps.

What I did not know about until later was that Audrey had had a cyst on her left eyelid for four years. Her doctor had thought it might be skin cancer, but three specialists were unable to commit themselves and finally told her just to leave it alone. After her second visit for healing she noticed that the cyst had turned red. It then became a scab and eventually simply peeled off. The migraines she had previously suffered with, too, became a thing of the past.

I have found that many patients are reluctant to tell their doctors of the benefit they have derived from healing, even if orthodox medicine has failed them. Perhaps they feel guilty for having sought another kind of treatment, or fear being disbelieved or ridiculed. But thankfully there are now many more medical practitioners who are open to the work of genuine healers – and some who even insist that their patients go to one.

Healing is too important to be ignored. Even when a cure is not completely effected, healing often leads to an immensely improved quality of life and peace of mind. I would like to see some serious long-term research carried out into the phenomenon of healing and have long striven for this. I look at it this way: if a new drug helped only ten per cent of the people to whom it was given, large sums of money would be spent on research. Yet no research is being done on healing, despite the fact that it helps more than forty per cent of those who seek it.

Shaw. He had found that he was becoming increasingly short of breath – he was smoking approximately twenty cigarettes a day. Worried, he booked an appointment with his doctor who immediately admitted him to hospital. X-rays were taken and fluid drained from his lungs. A special 'sealant' was introduced into the lung to coat the area where the fluid had been entering. He was told that he had a malignant tumour. It was located in an inaccessible place, and as it had already begun to spread, surgery was not feasible.

Edward came to see me the following spring, on his sister's advice. He was not sure healing would be of use to him, but decided it was worth a try. At first he came every fortnight, then once a month, over a period of two years. From the various conversations we had, Edward found that he was starting to view things differently. He was able to start believing in himself.

Attending for his regular check-up at the hospital, Edward was told by the doctors that the tumour had gone and that he need not go back again.

Were it not for the hospital's early action, Edward feels things might not have turned out so well. But he is also sure that without healing the tumour would still be on his lung. 'Never give in' he says. 'Fight it all the way. Healing comes from a positive attitude.'

It was this same positive attitude that helped another patient, a woman of eighty-three who was suffering with throat cancer. She was due to have surgery on the left side of her throat to remove her voice box, but decided not to go ahead with the operation. Radiotherapy treatment had not worked and by the time of her second visit for healing, the cancer had spread to her tongue. I did not see her again for several months, but by this time a specialist at the Marsden Hospital had told her that the cancer was dormant. She came for healing several more times. The cancer recurred for a while, but a few months later, the specialist was puzzled to find that it no longer seemed to be progressing. My patient was able to enjoy life again, eating and drinking without pain.

5

The Cancer Patient

Experience is not what happens to you; it is what you
do with what happens to you.

Aldous Huxley

Cancer sufferers, research has shown, are people who think
too little of themselves. It does not always show, but it is
always there – a classic kind of dis-ease connected with a
particular kind of disease. I always tell my patients that
they need to practise being a little kinder to themselves.
Martin Israel put it something like this: 'The very fact that
the Guv'nor went to all the trouble to put such a living miracle
as YOU together in the first place, makes it quite clear that –
being omnipotent and omniscient as He is – He surely loved
you enough to do it.' So, whether you like it or not, you are
loved anyway. If you understand this, it becomes easier to
live that 'specialness' you already are. If only one person ever
honestly says 'I love you' your whole life has been worthwhile.
Perhaps the great wonder about this is that so often people are
loved by many rather than just one other.

Our bodies in fact make cancer cells all the time, but
normally the immune system can identify them and so
destroy them. If the immune system is not working as
well as it might, the cancer cells start making a nuisance
of themselves. When we are tense or anxious rather than
relaxed, the 'kit' cannot work as well as it should. If this
state of stress goes on long-term, so that we are preventing
a part of our body working as it should, something is bound
to go wrong.

One patient who came for healing for cancer was Edward

Everything starts in the mind. The drug revolution that has taken off since the war is now proving not to be the magic answer doctors had once thought, with drugs often causing more problems than answers. Many people come to a healer as a last resort, when drugs have not worked. But there are now an increasing number who come to a healer first, rather than to a doctor. However, I always ask my patients 'What does your doctor say about it?', strongly advising them to seek medical advice if they are not already doing so. I know some healers who actually tell their patients that they should not see a doctor! This is both ridiculous and dangerous and I would certainly never interfere in any way between a patient and his or her medical treatment.

Making use of healing has much to do with how the patient happens to think – and how the patient thinks may usefully change. It is not the patient being persuaded to think as the healer thinks, for the healer can only tell the patient the best he knows without pretending that what he thinks is the best there is.

There are two good places for a patient to start to help himself. They are things for him to think about so that he may find an increase of inner tranquillity or ease – *ease* is the opposite of *dis-ease*. The patient playing *his* part in healing could be described as promoting or increasing *ease* within that part of him which is not the physical body.

The first thing to consider is that you are *not* your body. You have a body, but it is not something you are, it is simply something you have. You and your body are two different things that happen to be involved with each other, and that is called 'living in the world'. Your body is made of material – flesh and blood – and *you* are *not*.

There are plenty of things that are not made of material, but are none the less real. 'Thought', 'love' and 'art' are just three of them. These things sometimes find expression in or through material but do not depend upon material to exist – as with the thought that had to happen before the chair you are sitting on existed. Exactly the same applies to you. The churches say that you are a body with a soul. But a soul is

not something that you have – it is something that you *are*.
The body is not something you are – it is something you have.
It is therefore better to understand that you are a *soul with
a body*.

So what is real is *you*, the part which is not made of material
but which inhabits and animates the body. And because, as I
explained, your body is ninety per cent space, you may see
that it is less solid, less dense than you might have thought. It
is therefore also more subject to change than you might have
thought – just as cooking oil melts quicker than candle grease
because its density is less. Any healing process is a matter of
beneficial changes taking place. Getting sick is change in the
other direction.

Add one other ingredient – the one and only constant in life
– the fact that everything changes all the time. A brick wall
is changing all the time even though it does not appear to be
changing. One day it will crumble away. The great difference
between your body and the brick wall is that the brick wall
has no choice about change and you do.

If you understand the above you can never suppose that
you can't get better – no matter what anyone says. What you
can say is, 'I can get better, I can get worse – but I cannot
stay the same.' And what is more, you have a lot of choice in
the matter. Of course, you don't have to do it all by yourself;
the power of healing can help you and so can other things,
including science. It all depends on the use you can make of
the treatment. I use the word '*can*' rather than '*will*', simply
because I am a healer and not a fortune-teller.

The second thing to consider is that anything which is
unique is, by definition, totally special. *You* are unique – so
when did you last think of yourself as *totally special*? If you do
not, it is high time you started doing so, because it is true.

Just as you and your body are two different things, so
what you do and what you are anyway are two different
things. Whatever happens to you does not alter the fact that
you are unique. What happens may or may not make you
comfortable, but it does not change the fact: you are still
unique, and therefore totally special.

What anyone else thinks of you alters it not one bit and we are back again to the man with half a bottle of wine. It does not matter what you think, none of this destroys compassion or morality. But when we forget these things we are hurting ourselves.

It is not being conceited to think of yourself as totally special, because – know it or not – so is everyone else.

It may help to consider how it came about in the first place that you are unique. I have no particular religion, but I do know one thing for sure – you can't have design without there being a designer. Look at a rose – or all creation – it is marvellous design at work. We muck it up all the time; but of itself, it is all marvellous design. It is surely a matter of common sense that what you may think of as 'God' or 'The Creator' or what I call 'The Guv'nor' exists. This is enough for me, without worrying myself as to whether He is a Catholic, or a Muslim, or whatever.

There is nothing wrong with *you* for, as distinct from your body, *you* are *totally special*. You started out *totally special*. You can't improve on 'totally special'. You can ignore it, or lose sight of it, but you can't lose it. *You* are permanent and all the rest is experience through which you have, for a while, the opportunity to learn whatever you need or want to learn. The adventure of *being* never comes to an end. It is just the scenery which keeps changing.

Many world religions say 'God is Love'. What they do not seem to understand is that therefore 'Love is God'. Everyone has some love within him. Love is not rationed but we are inclined to ration it, and that is not compulsory. So you have within you the power that created the whole universe. And to get well and stay that way, why not try using some of it on yourself. You may then see that, whatever ails you, you are not quite the victim you thought you were.

It was having a positive attitude – the urge to fight back – that one of my patients feels was responsible for her recovery from cancer. This is her story:

I have written about my experience of cancer in the hope that it might help others to gain ideas about fighting the disease.

In June 1987 it was discovered that I had breast cancer and needed a complete mastectomy. This was done at the Royal Marsden Hospital, Sutton and it was decided there was no need for radiotherapy or chemotherapy. I was put on the drug Tamoxifen and all went well for two years until I noticed little nodules appearing along the scar where the breast had been removed. The Marsden decided to change my drugs and keep an eye on the nodules so I was making regular visits to the hospital.

When I realized the cancer had returned, I felt I needed to try to seek extra help. I had heard of a healer living in Sussex who had helped a friend of mine, so I decided to go and see him. I must admit I was very sceptical as to whether he could really help me as I could not understand how such things could 'work'.

My first visit to Phil was a week before a visit to the Marsden where they wanted to have another look at the three nodules. The first question when they looked at the nodules was 'where is the third nodule?'. One had completely disappeared. I continued with treatment at the Marsden and I kept up my visits to Phil. I told the Marsden I was visiting a healer.

During our talks, one thing Phil made me understand was that our body is just a vehicle; that when we die we discard this vehicle and our soul, our mind (whatever we call it) carries on. He made me realize that I am in control of my own body on this earth and that if I did not want cancer then I could decide to rid myself of it. I confessed during one talk that although I was not afraid of dying, I was very much afraid of the *way* in which I might die and concerned as to who would have the bother of looking after me. Phil told me there was no need for *me* to worry about that – when the time came there would be someone to look after me.

Gradually, however, the cancer seemed to worsen. In

fact I was told it had spread to the spine, and eventually the Marsden suggested I should start chemotherapy. I had always dreaded this as I felt it could not *cure* cancer but only enabled you to live a little longer, but with possible bad side-effects, and I felt quality of life was more important than quantity. Reluctantly, however, I agreed and I had my first and only dose on Friday, 19th April, 1991. The reaction was dramatic and on the Thursday, 25th April, I was taken to the Princess Alice Hospice at Esher. The nurses told me afterwards that I was in such a terrible state they did not expect me to live the night through. I certainly did not want to live. I could eat nothing, could only manage a sip of water, my mouth was full of sores and thrush and I had to be lifted by nurses to sit or lie down in the bed. My hair was falling out rapidly and I could not be bothered with anything.

The hospice is a wonderful place, with a happy, caring atmosphere. It is impossible to praise the staff too highly. Gradually, very gradually, they persuaded me to try a spoonful or two of their home-made soup, then it was a little rice pudding or ice cream. Nothing was too much trouble for them and they appeared to have endless time to spend with one. My family and friends rallied round, someone came to see me every day. My mother, aged 92, always came, brought by different friends or helpers of the hospice. All this time Phil Edwardes gave me absent healing. But something was not right. I was given all this wonderful support and love, yet my own will to live had gone. I was hardly aware of it at the time, but I remember each time my son came he tried to urge me to fight, to get back the old 'spark'.

I have tried so hard to understand what it was that brought back my desire to live, as I felt this is the important thing for others in my position to understand. Of course we are all different and what works for one may not work for others, but what worked for me may help others to try.

One morning I was watching the patient opposite me as staff were trying to get her to take a few steps with a walking frame. She was not interested, although they tried for several days, until she refused to attempt it any more. I then thought to myself: 'I'm sure I could try that – it would be wonderful to be able to move by myself, albeit with the help of a frame.' I was still needing the help of two nurses to go anywhere. I asked if I could try the frame and they immediately sent for the physiotherapist. It took me all my willpower to do two steps – but it was a start.

The physiotherapist and the staff were wonderful and encouraged me for all they were worth, making a considerable joke of it: '. . . we'll have you tearing down those corridors soon . . . .' I got the nickname 'Speedo', although in actual fact I was crawling everywhere. However, I gradually improved by setting myself a new target each day – say to a certain point down a corridor and the next day a little bit further. Then one day I had used the frame to get to the bathroom, was in the bath, and the nurse said to me, 'What is your aim for today?' I said, half jokingly, 'I'd love to be able to walk back to my bed without the frame.' To my surprise she said 'Go on then, let's see you do it.' She was careful to walk very closely behind me, but I did it.

Now the point of all this is to show that what brought me back to wanting to live was to have a series of aims or goals. I did not do it deliberately or have a definite plan worked out – I took each day as it came and had not even considered that I might get better and leave the hospice. I just had to have a challenge for that day and through doing this, and achieving the challenge, I was keeping a positive attitude to everything. If I did not achieve the challenge that day, then I worked at it until I *did*.

Another way I helped myself was by visualizing. There are all manner of ways in which you can do this – imagine knights on horses charging the cancer cells and killing them. Imagine the sun's rays reaching into your body from the head to the feet and burning out all the cancer cells – you will find a way that suits you best.

A further thing I found helpful was to deliberately relax. It is quite hard to learn but once you've learnt you can put it into practice any time. I used to think myself back into Phil Edwardes' healing room. Phil told me to remember that cancer is dis-ease, and to help fight it you need to be relaxed in yourself – not all tense and stressed. There are various relaxation tapes that can help you.

One thing that seems incredible to me on looking back is that I did not ever realize I had lung cancer. I should have realized when I went into the hospice that something serious must have happened but I seemed quite incapable of thought then. The last time I went to the Marsden they showed me the X-ray of my lungs and they were completely clear, yet the X-ray from the year before showed one lung full of cancer. The doctor at the Marsden called me 'a walking miracle' as they had given me three months to live when I came out of the hospice – that was nearly a year ago.

The main thing towards helping yourself, I am convinced, is to have a set of goals. I still do it now as it is vital to keep on top of this disease. I find it useful to have goals for different periods – daily, weekly, monthly and yearly. A very useful book for this is *Getting Well Again* by O. Carl Simonton and published by Bantam Books.

I have had marvellous support from family and friends. I have a healer in whom I firmly believe and who I know has played a major role in my recovery. I have had physical help from the Marsden and mental help from the hospice, but I must stress that it is largely down to the individual in the end. Keep a positive attitude in your thinking, set and reach your goals, and you will beat cancer.

How is it that babies and young children may become seriously ill, perhaps with cancer, even though they have not had time to experience the stresses of life that cause disease? I would explain it like this: at the moment of your birth, you and your body come together – which could not happen if they had not existed separately before this. In other words, you always have existed and you always will. All your experience is indelibly recorded in your subconscious mind, and in hypnosis you can be taken back – sometimes to the time before you were born, for instance in your mother's womb, or to the moment of your birth: who was present at the time, what was said. You can also be taken back to a time before you were conceived – who and where you were, whether it was on this earth or in another existence. Anyone's character, at any one time, is the sum total of the use they have made of their experience.

When a child is born it comes into the world with its own character – which is unique – and despite the genetic circumstances of its birth and the attitudes of the family in which it is brought up, schooling and so on, that child is still an individual in its own right. When we say 'This child is only five', what we mean is that the child has only lived in this world for five years. The fact is that we are ageless. A hundred years may seem a long time, but the reality is that there is no difference between five minutes and a thousand years – because it is always now. YOU ARE and always will be. And we are all part of one another – we cannot blame one specific person for an ailment, but would have to take everyone else in the world into consideration when apportioning blame!

Not only are all diseases caused, in one way or another, by stress, they are also hereditary – we make ourselves ill and that illness, if not recognized and dealt with as a 'lack of ease', is carried on through others.

Kelly was three and a half years old when she was brought for healing by her grandfather. Doctors had diagnosed a cancerous brain cyst. Kelly took to the healing at once, describing it as 'tickly'. Her mother later said that Kelly had been aware that something 'good' was happening to her head during the healing and she very quickly got back some of the mobility in her right arm and leg, which had been badly affected by the tumour.

Shortly afterwards, Kelly began radiation treatment at Guy's Hospital in London. Her mother told the Professor in charge of her case that she was taking her daughter for healing and his response was encouraging: 'We do not know what healers can do, but it is worth a try.' Radiation was given for five days a week and Kelly would then come back for an appointment with me at the week-end. It was noticeable that after the cyst was drained at the hospital, no painkillers were needed. She always recovered remarkably quickly, too, from the radiotherapy, with none of the usual side-effects. The hospital were very pleased with her progress.

Three months later Kelly began to suffer with a severe pain in her right side. After healing the pain vanished. Soon she was eating and sleeping better and her right-hand facility had greatly improved. When Kelly came back for healing a week later and asked to sit on the stool on her own, her mother was worried. She knew how tired Kelly always felt after healing and wondered if she would fall asleep and topple off the stool. So she sat with Kelly on her lap. Although Kelly was a lot better by this time, her mother was still rather sceptical about healing and had more faith in the hospital treatment she was receiving. But she said that as soon as I started passing my hands over Kelly's head she knew it was real. The tingling sensation her daughter had often described passed right through her. She says she feels sad that, although she has friends with children who are not responding to medical treatment, they will not take them for healing. She has told them about her own experiences but has not been able to convince them.

Kelly continued to make good progress. Four months later she had a brain scan. The first reports looked encouraging and the results read 'Tumour is shrinking'.

Although she has not yet recovered full use of her right arm and leg, Kelly has become stronger and livelier. Her mother describes her as a determined child with a fighting spirit, who is not afraid to tackle anything new. She has learnt to ski and is becoming a very proficient swimmer. Further medical tests have all revealed good progress. Of the five children in her hospital ward – all suffering with cancer – Kelly was the only survivor. She was also the only child having healing.

Even with the most serious illness, there are no limits to the possible beneficial changes that may be brought about by healing. A teenage boy who had had two major operations for a malignant soft-tissue sarcoma on his thigh was introduced to healing by his mother. The surgeon had discovered that the cancer had spread to both the boy's lungs and he could not give any real hope for his recovery. Tests showed that five and a half months of intensive chemotherapy had had no effect on the tumours, but they had remained stable and so could be removed. This, the patient's mother is convinced, is due to the healing he received during that time. He has now gone on to university, and feels confident about the future.

The medical profession discovered that when you laugh your brain makes chemicals which your body needs. The same thing happens when there is sunlight. It is also known that when you are angry your stomach lining becomes inflamed. Your mind is the bridge between you and your brain. The brain is the tool of the mind and the body is the tool of the brain. *You* are in charge of all of it. So, making use of healing could be described as you using something you already have – your mind – to more fully *realize* something else which is already true: there is nothing wrong with *you*, it is only the body that may ail.

It is mostly a matter of 'allowing'. A good healer should allow healing to occur rather than try to 'do' it. A patient should allow the body to heal or, better still, allow himself to '*be*' what he really is: '*totally special*'. This allows the power he really is to flood his being. Healing power then reinforces it.

Valerie Wellings, a speech therapist in her fifties, found that coming for healing produced a dramatic change in her outlook. She had felt anxious and fearful when cancer was again diagnosed after nine problem-free years. Her feeling of relaxation and confidence increased with subsequent visits and she says that sharing a joke helped in the healing process – 'It was my mental state I was battling with'.

A malignant melanoma, in the form of an enlarged mole, had been removed from her left shin bone nine years before. She was shocked when there was a second, followed by a third recurrence of the problem. First she noticed a nodule in the knee area which grew from the size of a pea to that of a broad bean within months. This was followed, six months later, by a similar type of nodule that was developing on the original scar. Her confidence was shattered and she immediately began worrying about her family, imagining the effect on them should her fears be realized.

Valerie says 'I know I shall always remember the contrast of how I felt before and after my first visit. I was very up-tight initially, but came away a different person. My family quickly noticed the change in me.' She made three subsequent visits, at weekly intervals, and describes a sense of total relaxation during healing. 'Everything just left me. I remember sitting there with my hands tightly clasped at first, but by the end all the tension had gone out of them.'

My patient also consulted a herbalist and felt that the two therapies together gave her a positive attitude, the feeling that she could help herself – something, she says, that doctors do not always inspire. A change of diet, cutting out junk food, has also helped.

Now, there is no sign of the nodules that had caused Valerie so much worry. She feels she will always want to come back for healing once in a while, for the encouragement and support it gives her. And she says she would recommend it to anyone, knowing how very low she was feeling beforehand. 'No-one should discount it.'

Healing cannot be imposed upon anyone. It is only offered, like anything else that may be offered. The use of it may depend upon what use the patient may be able to make of it. Healing cannot be imposed, because of where it originates from. 'Love itself never insists' – only we do that. Sai Baba*

* Sai Baba is an avatar and teacher who lives in India and has great influence for good throughout the world.

tells a lovely story about a man who was very religious and who attended church with great regularity. He couldn't swim and he fell in the river. He prayed very hard to God to save him and was sure he had been heard. Someone threw him a rope, which he rejected, saying 'I don't need that, for God will save me'. Someone else threw him a life belt, which he also rejected. Two men arrived in a rowing boat and got the same rejection. Then he drowned. When he reached The Guv'nor, he asked 'Did you not hear me?' The Guv'nor said 'Of course I did. I sent you a man with a rope, another with a life belt and two more in a rowing boat. But you took no notice.'

I AM THERE
(by James Dillet Freeman)

Do you need Me? I AM there.
You cannot see Me, yet I AM the Light you see by.
You cannot hear Me, yet I speak through your voice.
You cannot feel Me, yet I AM the Power at work in your hands.

I AM at work, though you do not understand My ways.
I AM at work, though you do not understand My works.
I AM not strange visions; I AM not mysteries.
Only in absolute stillness, beyond self, can you know Me as
    I AM – and then but as a feeling and a faith.

Yet I AM there. Yet I hear. Yet I answer.

When you need Me, I AM there.
Even if you deny Me, I AM there.
Even when you feel most alone, I AM there.
Even in your fears, I AM there.
Even in your pain, I AM there.
I AM there when you pray, and when you do not pray.

I AM in you, and you are in Me.
Only in your mind can you feel separate from Me,
For only in your mind are the mists of 'yours' and 'mine'.
Yet only with your mind can you know Me and experience Me.

Empty your heart of empty fears.
When you get yourself out of the way, I AM there.
You can of yourself do nothing, but I can do all,
And I AM in all.

Though you may not see the good, good is there, for I AM there.

I AM there because I have to be, because I AM.
Only in Me does the world have meaning;
Only out of Me does the world take form;
Only because of Me does the world go forward;
I AM the Law on which the movement of the stars and the
    growth of living cells are founded.
I AM the Love that is the Law's fulfilling.
I AM Assurance.
I AM Peace.

I AM ONENESS.
I AM the Law that you can live by.
I AM the Love that you can cling to.
I AM your assurance.
I AM your peace.
I AM ONE with you.
I AM.

Though you fail to find Me, I do not fail you.
Though your faith in Me is unsure, My faith in you never
    wavers —
Because I KNOW YOU, because I LOVE YOU.

Beloved, I AM there.

(A copy of *I Am There* is now on the moon — taken there on
the Apollo XV voyage by astronaut James B. Irwin.)

6

When Healing Seems To Fail

Though you fail to find Me, I do not fail you.
Though your faith in Me is unsure, My faith in you
  never wavers –
Because I KNOW YOU, because I LOVE YOU.
Beloved, I AM there.

Healing is for the *whole* person. If the spirit is not touched I would not consider healing a success – because true healing is for the spirit. A healer does no healing, but simply allows it, which the patient needs to do also. If healing fails, I believe it is because the sufferer cannot, for whatever reason, accept it. A healer does not need to know the physiological details of what is wrong with a patient. I once spoke to a very insistent young newspaper reporter who could not understand how anyone could get better if I did not know exactly what was wrong with them. I made the mistake of explaining that I honestly would not know the difference between a hernia and a jock-strap. He printed this remark, which may have lowered the tone a bit, but is nevertheless true! I make notes of the patient's description of his condition at the start only as a point of reference for the future, to see how things may change.

Very early in my healing work a man came with two separate points of pain in the spine – one at the base and one between the shoulder blades. He had suffered with the condition for many years and had been told that he would just have to live with it as nothing more could be done. On his second visit I asked him how he was and he said that he was no better. He then described at length the pain at the base of the spine but said nothing about the higher pain. When I mentioned it he exclaimed with surprise that he had had no pain there since his last visit. He had completely forgotten the pain of all those years – and rightly so. If you have a headache you know it. When it is gone you do not want to 'know' it and it is best forgotten. I could not help asking 'What was that you were saying about being no better?' There is a difference between what we want and what we need. Through healing we receive what we really need, which may or may not be what we want. This is why some are healed more quickly than others – why some are healed when others are not.

Even if healing does not bring about a lasting physical cure, it will often bring peace of mind that comes from a deeper understanding. Peter Liddall had contracted cancer a year before he came to see me. Doctors had initially pronounced his condition to be inoperable. And yet after three visits, within one month, for healing, the hospital scan showed the tumour to be virtually arrested – which his specialist said was 'against expectation'. The stability continued. It was even suggested that the tumour might be diminishing. Doctors were puzzled that Peter appeared to be getting better, despite all their previously gloomy predictions. Peter was a charming man, and a fighter. It was that spirit which, no doubt, contributed to his living for another year – considerably longer than had originally been envisaged. The night before his first operation, Peter wrote the following poem.

REFLECTION
(In a Different Light)

When you are far away from your fellow man
  with only the sounds of the night
Does your heart reach out for the truth about life
  and your spirit cry for what's right?

You are rushing along like a wave in a storm
  no purpose or target in view

You curse any man who gets in your way
  without any thought of his due.

The next time you pause and look at the sky,
  take a moment to ponder alone –
everyone in this world, indeed and beyond
  has an ego that's just like your own

Could it be that that spark, that consciousness part,
  which everyone has at his birth
Is one and the same, a mere spark from a flame,
  from a source that is not of this earth.

So next time you're vexed with the person you're next
  be he black, be he yellow or white;
look beyond that thin skin to the soul that's within
  for it's you in a different light.

Peter died nearly two years later. Healing had in the end not
cured his cancer. But a close friend wrote 'It is very significant
that Adele, his wife, has always maintained that healing did so
much for Peter, for it helped in the most important manner –
it gave her husband peace of mind.'

This reading, by an unknown author, was given at the
morning cremation service:

FOOTPRINTS

One night a man had a dream. He dreamt he was
walking along the beach with the Lord. Across the sky
flashed scenes from his life. For each scene, he noticed
two sets of footprints in the sand. One belonging to
him, the other to the Lord. When the last scene of his
life flashed before him, he looked back at the footprints
in the sand. He noticed that many times along the path
of his life there was only one set of footprints. He also
noticed that it happened at the very lowest and saddest
times in his life.

This really bothered him and he questioned the Lord about it. Lord, you said that once I decided to follow you, you would walk with me all the way. But I have noticed that during the most troublesome times in my life, there is only one set of footprints. I do not understand why, when I needed you most, you would leave me.

The Lord replied: My son, my precious child, I love you and would never leave you. During your times of trial and suffering, when you see only one set of footprints, it was then that I carried you.

A doctor writing on the subject of healing could not understand, and considered a 'nonsense statement', the following reaction of a blind man who had sought healing: 'I maintain that I have been healed, though my blindness has not been taken away – because I have been lifted above it and it has become no handicap to me. I am healed.'

That healing exists there can be no doubt. But our understanding of it is by no means complete. I see no need for anything but a simple approach, with no fuss or ceremony, and plenty of humour. But I also feel strongly that, with more research and therefore greater knowledge, we may well find better methods of approach and therefore increased success.

Fear has a direct bearing on recovery from illness. A negative outlook will work against healing. I have found that those with a positive approach usually get better more quickly. Some people come for healing once or twice and are never heard of again. Perhaps their problem has been eased, and they presume that I will be aware of this without their telling me. But there are also those who, not having experienced immediate or lasting benefit, consider that healing has failed and they do not come back for this reason.

YOU are in charge of your body. It is not in charge of you, even if that seems to be the case. Healing cannot be imposed upon anyone, but is a matter of co-operation between the patient and the source of healing power – which is *not* the healer. That which we ARE merely inhabits the body.

Recovery can quite often be a 'slow but sure' process, requiring persistence from the patient. Lesley had been involved in two car accidents that left her with severe whiplash, wrecking the mechanics of her spine. Physiotherapy had proved of no use, and although a cranial osteopath had been able to help restore the mobility of her spine, Lesley started to look around for other methods of treatment that might be able to help. She contacted the healer Matthew Manning in Suffolk, and he was able to help ease her neck. But after several visits, she decided to come to Roundstreet for treatment, as this was a shorter distance from her home. Lesley found that healing was of most benefit if she came regularly and did not leave long gaps between visits. Unfortunately, when travelling with a friend who was forced to brake sharply, she was again left with whiplash and further aggravation of the damage. But with regular and reasonably frequent visits for healing, she is making steady progress.

It can happen that patients will decide not to continue with healing as soon as they experience some beneficial change, even though I advise them to come back. By the time Jenny's cancer had been diagnosed by doctors, they told her she had just three months to live. No medical treatment was available for her particular type of cancer and she was in despair. She came for healing and reported being 'bombarded with coloured lights' during the session. She came once a week, for a month, before going back to Guy's Hospital for her usual check-up. At the hospital she was told that she was cured and could go back to work. Delighted, Jenny rang me to tell me the news, but I told her she must continue coming for healing. She declined. She had believed the doctors when they told her she was 'cured' and was so pleased to be working again and living a normal life, she wanted to forget all about the cancer. I felt so worried, I telephoned her at home and also rang a relative of hers, so strongly did I feel that Jenny should come back to see me. But despite all the arguments and attempts at pursuasion, Jenny would not agree. She went for a week's holiday with some colleagues from work and returned home with a cough. Sadly, within a few weeks she had been admitted to a hospice and not long afterwards she died.

Generally speaking, symptoms are the body's way of letting us know that all is not well. Sometimes after healing they may temporarily worsen, but this can be a positive sign that things are improving. Margaret had suffered with a painful back problem for forty years. At the age of seventeen a fall had resulted in damage to the lower spine. In latter years the dorsal and cervical spine also began to give out. She had attended a London specialist for some years, and he had tried various forms of manipulation and injections. But he had also told her that he could do no more than keep the condition temporarily in check. He could not reverse it.

After her first visit, Margaret asked me if I had been massaging her neck. I assured her I would never do this, as it might aggravate the damage. Yet she reported a very strong sensation of someone forcefully digging their thumbs into both sides of her neck, at the top of her spine. She also had a great feeling of warmth and well-being. When she got home she switched on the television, planning to watch a film. But she never saw it because she uncharacteristically fell fast asleep in her chair. Within a week, Margaret noticed a great improvement in the condition of her back.

But after her second visit, Margaret was one day in the bathroom, preparing to go out with her husband, when she suddenly felt 'the most excruciating pain' in the dorsal area of her spine, between the shoulder blades. 'I sat on the side of the bath and went through the most unbelievable spasms of pain. Two hours later, however, it just felt sore. Then a couple of hours after that I felt marvellous – almost completely without pain.' The improvement in her condition has continued, the only set-backs occurring if she over-confidently lifts too heavy a weight. The pain she had suffered for most of her life is now much reduced and she has not been back to her specialist since.

More often than not, healing is a matter of 'two steps forward, one step back', and it is sad when patients who do not see dramatic and lasting results feel that healing has failed and do not persevere with their treatment. Or they forget or begin to doubt the benefit they felt.

Jamie Coad was twelve when he began complaining that his feet hurt. Day after day, for three weeks, he came home from school crying with the pain. Wendy, his mother, thought at first that he was just playing up. But it soon became obvious that there really was something wrong and she took Jamie to the hospital for a check-up. What the doctors found came as a great shock. Unknown to her, she had a very rare bone disorder, causing 'calcaneous bars' which, it turned out, she had passed on to both her children. The bones in Jamie's feet were slowly but surely welding together. The disorder had already slightly affected Wendy in her spine but her son's problem was far more severe. The doctors said they would have to operate. Wendy took Jamie to the chiropractor she had been seeing for her own back trouble. He was unable to help. Other 'alternative' practitioners also proved unsuccessful and she was beginning to feel desperate.

Jamie was not very enthusiastic at the idea of going to a healer, thinking it would be a waste of time. But he said afterwards that he had had the sensation of a tremendous tugging at his ankles while he was sitting on the stool in the healing room. He felt he had to pull himself backwards to stop himself falling off. He wondered if I was doing the tugging until he realized my hands were still moving over his back. The tugging became so strong that he began to hope I would be able to hold him steady and stop him falling off the stool altogether!

The week before I saw Jamie had been a particularly bad one for him. The pain had been so severe that he had hardly been able to walk. With the bones slowly locking together, he could no longer bend his feet and was only able to move along in a stooped, flat-footed shuffle. So when Wendy saw her son walk quite normally out of the healing room, she could hardly believe her eyes. She was also amazed at the improvement in her son's personality afterwards. An aggressive child before, because of the pain and lack of mobility – he would kick things across the kitchen in his frustration – he became again the gentle son she had previously known. He came three more times, over the next two months, and Wendy felt that not only her son's symptoms were eased, but that he was helped as a whole: mind, body and spirit.

Not long afterwards a letter arrived from the hospital with the date for his first operation. The 'welded' condition of the bones in Jamie's feet still appeared unchanged and it seemed sensible to accept whatever treatment was available. The surgeon was to operate on one foot at a time. In order to make room for the foot to move, large chunks of bone were removed from the ankle. He was in plaster for six months afterwards, as well as a good deal of pain. Only one month after the plaster was removed, Jamie had to go through the whole ordeal again, this time with the other foot. A third operation, to weld the bones in his ankles and feet together to stop them crumbling away, was cancelled indefinitely due to NHS cutbacks.

So why has Jamie not come back for healing since those four visits he made before the operations? Wendy says he feels he has to give the bones time to settle down – that he has resigned himself to the pain after such major surgery and because the disease is said to be incurable. Yet he had been 'absolutely amazed' at what happened during and after the first healing. And he had continued to benefit from subsequent visits, both physically and mentally.

As has already been stated: healing cannot be imposed, it can only be *offered*. Progress may seem slow in coming. Instant and dramatic improvement after healing does happen, but time and perseverence is often needed. A riding accident left Linda Titheridge with loss of memory, pain in the left side of her head, neck and shoulder and tingling and weakness in her left arm and leg. Her balance was affected, she had double vision and could not look down, left or right. In addition her sense of taste and smell was damaged. During her second visit for healing Linda's head pain disappeared. Since her fourth visit she has had no problems with her balance and can now turn her head. Afterwards, single vision was restored for a couple of hours. Then, after her fifth visit, Linda experienced severe pain in her head, shoulder, neck, arm and leg, although the pain had cleared by the following day. I had to remind her that beneficial change is not always comfortable! Linda began to remember incidents from her past after her seventh visit for healing – the first time she had remembered anything that had happened before the accident. But she also found that she was sleeping badly again. Single-vision was restored temporarily after subsequent healing sessions and she eventually found she no longer needed sleeping pills.

Healing for Linda has been a gradual process, sometimes with no obvious improvement for a while. But she says that, apart from the specific improvements that have come about, she is feeling happier in general and is able to think more positively about herself and her future. She is still attending for healing sessions.

Healing is, most importantly of all, for the spirit – for the whole, essential person. Although physical problems may persist, as they did for Kieron Winn, healing can, nevertheless, be of benefit in an unexpected and fundamental way. Kieron sought healing for ear trouble, and this is his own account of his experience:

With encouragement from his son, I went to Phil with some persistent ear, nose and throat problems which the National Health Service was finding very hard to pin down. I was quickly put at ease during our initial chat. Phil very pursuasively argued the stress-related nature of illness, and that the only way to get better is from inside, from the self. To stay healthy one must be kind to oneself, which means not overloading one's diary and refusing to play too many games with the fools and madmen of this world. Principal among these he numbers most agents of established religions, which work through putting the fear of hell into people and suppressing too many of our natural instincts.

The main thing I felt during healing itself was a wonderful sense of reassurance, of everything suddenly being alright. It was like a thaw, or an immense and cleansing shiver, warm and cold at once, in which I convulsed a little, as if shaking something off. I have to emphasize how 'real' the experience was – however hard it may be to describe it satisfactorily, it most certainly was not any kind of private fantasy or desperate wish-fulfilment on my part. The sensations were completely overwhelming and as much physical as mental. Yet, despite the extraordinariness of those few minutes, everything I felt seemed so natural. Indeed I think of it now as a greatly amplified version of the effect of taking a few good, deep breaths – although I would not suggest that I could have felt as good without the healing. And perhaps this is the point: one of the best things Phil said was that nothing he could say or do would be anything more than a reminder of what all of us instinctively know, but tend to forget. Healing for me meant a restoration of the principle of health, a goal of well-being to bear in mind. For some time afterwards it was as if I was eight again and entirely unstressed. By being calmed so deeply, the world was set in order and it felt like coming home.

7

Bereavement

Death is nothing at all
I have only slipped away into the next room . . .

from *All Is Well* by Henry Scott Holland

This book is about healing, not clairvoyance or spiritualism or other aspects of the paranormal. But the following story of my son Phillip has been of help to so many of my patients that I am going to tell it here briefly. Some readers may find it hard to believe, but I am only setting down what actually happened as I and Sue experienced it.

As soon as Phillip had passed his seventeenth birthday he began asking me if he could have a more powerful motor-bike, a 250cc machine instead of the 50cc one he was using to get to work each day. I have always regarded motor-bikes as very dangerous and at first I resisted. I tried to persuade him to wait till he was eighteen and old enough to drive a car. But Phillip persisted and in the end I gave way. The boy had not had an easy time since his accident at nine years old and this motor-cycle would be an asset to him in his job.

The new machine came on a Friday in August. Phillip was delighted with it and wasted no time in trying it out.

The next day, Saturday, I was at the Gatwick garage with Sue. A message came through from the police. Phillip had had an accident and had been taken to hospital.

This time the doctors were optimistic. Phillip's leg had been broken and was in traction. There was some internal damage and his spleen would have to be removed. But his head had been protected by the helmet and there was no brain damage. When his mother and I got there he was sitting up in bed, fully conscious and reasonably comfortable. He was more concerned about the state of his motor-bike than about himself. He wanted to know how soon it could be got back on the road.

The police were mystified as to the cause of the accident. Phillip had come off his bike for no apparent reason and had hit two other cars before fetching up at the side of the road. There were no skid marks and the witnesses were baffled as to why he had crashed. No one else was hurt.

During the next six days he was in hospital I of course saw him frequently. There was no real cause for concern, the doctors said. He was recovering well. The only thing that worried me was that he kept on about that motor-bike. Could it be repaired? When could he get it back on the road again?

I said: 'It was a good thing, wasn't it, Phillip, that no one else was hurt in that accident?'

He looked at me for a moment, then said: 'Dad, let's talk about a car.'

The bike was never mentioned again.

Six days after the accident, Friday again, the phone rang late at night. It was the hospital. Suddenly and inexplicably, Phillip had died.

The news of Phillip's death was all the more of a shock for being unexpected. There was no sleep for us that night. The following morning we three were together at Roundstreet — myself and Sue, and Ann, Phillip's mother.

The hospital telephoned to ask if we'd come over to collect Phillip's effects. Neither Ann nor I could face it; the route led past the place where his accident had occurred. I asked Sue if she would go. Unlike us she had only the vaguest idea where Phillip had crashed.

It was a wet, rainy day. Driving back from the hospital, Sue saw a lad standing at the side of the road. She began to slow, thinking he was hoping for a lift. When she got nearer she saw that he was staring as if puzzled at the road. As she went past he looked up. The face was Phillip's. She slowed and stopped.

When she looked back the roadside was deserted, the figure had vanished.

Back at Roundstreet she questioned me about the location of the accident. It was exactly where she had seen Phillip. I checked all the details of her description, even to the electric transformer which she had seen at the spot and which up till then I had not noticed. Her story held good. We agreed to keep this extraordinary experience to ourselves, to tell nobody.

The fact that Sue had seen Phillip, or the etheric form of Phillip, tallied with my own conviction that a person's spirit is not extinguished by physical death. By September I had a strong desire to try and make some kind of contact with Phillip, wherever he was now. Friends advised me to go to see Jessie Nason, a sensitive with a gift for making contact with people who have died.

I will always remember the day I went to her flat in London. It was 13 October 1977. She was an affable, cheerful woman who proceeded to talk about the weather. She did not ask me why I had come to see her and I did not volunteer any information.

Suddenly, in the middle of a chat about everyday things, she stopped dead and gave me an odd look. 'Who is that young man standing beside you? No, don't tell me, he's your son.'

There followed a long conversation, which I will not repeat, with Jessie Nason acting as mouthpiece for Phillip. I could see no one else in the room. But she reproduced Phillip's exact intonation and phraseology and told me a lot of personal and trivial things about him. Some of these I was only able to verify when I got back home, but all were true. I was being told all these things, she said, to prove that I really was in touch with Phillip.

Much of what she said was very comforting to me. Phillip had shown her a road, Jessie said, and told her that he had died in hospital. It would not have happened unless he had insisted on something and I was not to blame myself. He'd been supposed to go when he was nine, but had been given a second chance.

He also said, Jessie told me, that Sue had seen him since

he'd died. I knew that neither Sue nor I had mentioned this to a living soul.

Here was a complete stranger telling me about matters which were only known inside my most intimate family circle. But what I found most comforting was the impression I had of Phillip's happiness and contentment.

In the car outside I made careful notes while my memory was fresh. I intended to check every detail to see if I could fault Jessie Nason. I drove home with feelings of great peace and gratitude.

That was not the end of it. All the checking of details simply confirmed what Jessie had said. The best way I could think of expressing my gratitude was to ask her down to spend a day in the country with us. It was some months before she was able to take me up on my offer.

We walked round the garden and then went indoors for some tea. We were all sitting talking when she said: 'Your boy is with us now. He's standing over there by the fireplace.'

Later she relayed a piece of information which was totally unexpected. 'Your eldest daughter is moving house.'

'No, she's not,' I said. Teresa lived thirty miles away and we were daily ringing each other up.

'Oh, but she is,' Jessie insisted. 'That's what Phillip's telling me.'

To settle the matter I went to telephone my daughter.

'Yes, Dad, we are moving house,' Teresa said.

'But why haven't you mentioned it?'

'We didn't want to tell anyone until the contracts were exchanged. We only exchanged today.'

When Jessie had gone Sue told me that she too had seen Phillip. Just his face and then only for a moment before it faded. It was not the face of the boy who had suffered brain damage, with its slightly bland expression, but Phillip as he *would* have been at the age of seventeen if the tractor had not run over him when he was nine.

After that I did not persist in trying to make contact with Phillip. I don't think one should combat bereavement in this way. One must turn to those still living in this world with an open and giving attitude. It is enough to know that there is a bond of love which is not broken by death.*

You cannot destroy material, only change it. If something is burned, not one atom of matter is lost – it is merely changed into gases and ashes. Even less can you destroy something not made of material anyway.

'You can't die for the life of you.' The end of a life in the world is not an end or a beginning – it is just a change in a person's experience of *being*, and even then it is only a change in the scenery, as your body is just part of the scenery. It is no good asking 'Where do I go when I die?' 'Where' is a material measurement. It would be as sensible as trying to assess how much love you could fit into a certain place or how much thought a matchbox might contain. The fact of your *being* matters more to those who love you than where you happen to be. If this was not so, those who love you would love you less the further you were from them. So you can never cease to *be*. You *do* have all eternity ahead of you. Equally, all those years ago when you got yourself born – when you collected the 'kit' you wander about in, somewhere in that process *you* and your body came together and you were born. This could not have happened unless those two things existed before they came together. You therefore have always existed and always will exist. The adventure of *being* and learning never ends. 'Always' is, to say the least, quite a long time. Does not this put 'being in the world' into its right perspective? It is really only for a while.

From this a big question arises – *why*?

The churches say we are here to be tested. According to them, if you are good you get a pair of wings, and if not, you've 'had it'. So according to them The Creator is running some sort of silly competition for mankind – His own creation! If this is the case you have the perfect answer, which is to remind Him: 'You started it all'! What could He say?

* The material from the start of the chapter to here is condensed from *Healing for You* by Phil Edwardes and James McConnell, Thorsons, 1985.

I suggest another answer, which is simply that we are here to *learn* for a while. We are 'at school'. The only way one really learns anything is from practical experience. Theory is fine, but practice is often different and much more useful. If you look back on some of the traumas in your life you can often say 'I did not like that at the time, but maybe I learned something through it that I would not have learned any other way'.

I'm sure that you have noticed that no one in the world is perfect. Some people think they are, but really no one is. You don't go to school if you have learned all the lessons. You cannot have a one-sided coin, so the existence of opposites provides us with the scenario through which we may learn. If it were 'cotton wool and roses' all the way for all of us, no one would know it. There would be nothing with which to compare it.

It seems clear to me that we are 'at school', or at least, in one classroom or another of a 'great school' for a while. And in any school it is the best students who get into the sixth form, where they get the harder lessons. So if you feel that you have been to hell and back too often, it might help you to realize that this may say something very nice about you. You don't have to look for trouble, it will find you anyway! And after all, steel is forged in fire.

When a woman in her sixties came for healing for her arthritis she had at first been full of sadness at the loss of her beloved husband a few years before. She could not come to terms with the thought of never seeing him again. Her only son was living many miles away.

Then one day she told me about an experience she had had two weeks before. She had read in a newspaper that a medium was to give a demonstration of his 'sensitivity' in a town some distance from where she lived. She made up her mind to go, although her immediate worry was that she might meet someone she knew. However, as the meeting was several miles from her home, this seemed unlikely. She was careful not to tell anyone that she was going and to her relief there were no familiar faces in the audience when she arrived. She took her seat, not sure what to expect. The medium was a man who had come from Wales, someone of whom she had never heard before. During the course of his demonstration, he turned to her and said 'I have something to say to you – someone called Robert wants me to tell you how very happy he is that he was able to help Ian the other evening'. She had no idea what he could be talking about, except for the fact that her husband's name was Robert and her son's name was Ian.

She was due to telephone her son the following day, but decided to say nothing of the incident in case he thought she was 'potty'. But the first thing her son said to her was 'Mum, I'm lucky to be talking to you at all – and you are going to think I am potty when I tell you why'. It immediately struck her as strange that the same expression had passed through both their minds. She asked him what he meant and he explained: 'The other evening I was driving far too fast along a narrow lane when I suddenly heard Dad say 'For God's sake boy, slow down!' It was so real, he could have been right there in the car with me. So I did slow down. And around the next corner came one of those big American lorries on the wrong side of the road.'

At that moment, my patient told me, ninety-nine per cent of her sorrow and pain over her husband's death vanished, never to return. Because she had immediately realized several things: that her husband still existed, that he was aware of her and her son and still cared about them – and that one day she would see him again.

We must all die, but when you come to realize that the physical body is merely housing the eternal spirit, you start to see that death is not the end of life. It is simply a progression of the spirit. I often speak to patients who are grieving the loss of someone very close. I always remind them of certain facts they actually know but are not thinking about. The most devastating part of bereavement is when no one answers the question 'Where is the person I love? What has happened to them – will I ever see them again?' We begin to wonder about life, about death and what it is all about.

The official line from the churches, in my opinion, does not help at all, because the platitudes they come up with do not answer the questions we want answered. And the reason for this is that they do not know. When it begins to make sense to you that you are not your body – and you can't die for the life of you – then it becomes easier to cope with the grief of losing someone you love. But words are not enough – we need to feel the reality of our eternal selves. If the end of someone's life means the end of that person, then the whole of their life has been totally pointless. If you love someone you will know that their life is anything *but* pointless. So the logical conclusion must be that life cannot come to an end because it is not meaningless. The purpose of our existence does not cease with death.

You can find practical experience of your eternal self if you choose to look. Many people, though, will say 'There is nowhere to look' or worse 'You are not supposed to look'! Well, if I was going to live in New York I would want to know something about the place and I would make it my business to find out. The only true picture of New York is the one I would have once I actually got there, but this does not prevent me trying to find out about it beforehand.

The obvious way to find out something about what happens when we die – and this is the only certain thing we all face – is to go and see a good medium or 'sensitive' as I prefer to call them. We all have the power to listen in to ourselves, but this ability is more pronounced in a sensitive. For instance, there are plenty of people who play the violin, but only a few with the talent of Yehudi Menuhin!

How many times has it happened that, just as you are thinking of a friend you have not seen for months, he or she telephones. This demonstrates our own 'sensitivity' – but we are surprised when we hear from our friend because we have not learnt to unscramble the messages all around us – something the medium or sensitive is better able to do.

When we receive information, through a sensitive, that could only have come from the person whom we think is dead, we have to realize that he or she is, in fact, still with us. This realization can be the start of a whole new way of thinking. It is the so-called 'religious' who have always been worried by this seeking after knowledge – perhaps because it threatens their very existence. In the 1930s the Church of England appointed a panel of bishops to examine spiritualism. This they did exhaustively, resulting in two reports, one from the majority, one from the minority. The majority report came out in favour of what the spiritualists had found to be true. The report was then promptly suppressed! It was only finally published about ten years ago.

Anyone who is afraid of the truth of life should not set themselves up as 'moral' leaders of others. The religious hierarchy have a responsibility to their followers to be always open to truth. Because truth is a very important ingredient of love. If priests and bishops do not understand this, they are being disloyal to the very thing they profess to believe in.

Telepathy is thought of as a rare gift. But we all have it and use it constantly. During normal conversation thought is being passed from mind to mind. The means employed happen to be our voice and ears – and you will know that even these are not always necessary in a conversation with someone close to you.

In meditation (another word for prayer) we are asking questions of the Guv'nor and listening for the answers. I find that these answers are very often given in a way and at a time I had not expected. The ability to meditate – that is, sitting very quietly and listening – will be easier some days than others. That is why I have never seen the point in setting aside a specific time for meditation, as some suggest.

Inevitably there comes a time when we have to leave the 'kit' behind. But even if healing does not bring about a lasting physical cure, it has helped many patients find a great peace and calm during the last few months or years of their lives, and this can be of help and comfort to those left behind.

Captain Max Walker, OBE, had had a naval career distinguished by his having founded and commanded the Kenyan Navy in the years immediately following independence in 1963. When he was in his late fifties, Max was told that he had cancer of the pancreas. Surgeons carried out a by-pass operation the following month. He was told that he had about two years to live. The devastating news reduced his spirits to a very low ebb and his wife, Betty, began to look into the possibility of complementary therapies.

Two months later Max had recovered sufficiently from the surgery to travel to Bristol to the Cancer Help Centre. Here he learnt about relaxation and meditation and was also put on a special course of vitamins. Both Max's doctor and the Bristol Centre were encouraging on the subject of healers and he came to see me soon afterwards.

This was to be the first of many visits over the next three years. On this occasion Max arrived in very poor condition, both physically and mentally. Betty remembers how the healing, although undramatic at the time, always gave her husband a great sense of peace and relaxation, as well as lifting his spirits. Max continued with his treatment from the Cancer Help Centre, as well as a course of chemotherapy and radiation at the hospital. Three months after surgery he went back to full-time work and it became clear as time went on that he was going to outlive the doctors' predictions.

But three years on Max began to feel ill again. Betty wonders if the chemotherapy and radiation had been just too much for his system to cope with. His condition gradually worsened and a few months later he died.

Yet he had stayed well for longer than expected. Having received so many different types of therapy, Betty says she cannot be sure what exactly was working for him. But she says she knows the visits for healing gave Max a renewed sense of peace and a much more positive mental attitude. She believes it helped slow the cancer down so that his immune system could fight back and wonders whether more of this gentle treatment would have been better for him, instead of the chemotherapy. Betty was herself helped by healing when she was under stress and has found comfort in the message it carries.

A CREED
by John Masefield (1878–1967)

I hold that when a person dies
His soul returns again to earth;
Arrayed in some new flesh disguise,
Another mother gives him birth.
With sturdier limbs and brighter brain
The old soul takes the road again.

Such is my own belief and trust;
This hand, this hand that holds the pen,
Has many a hundred times been dust
And turned, as dust, to dust again;
These eyes of mine have blinked and shone
In Thebes, in Troy, in Babylon.

All that I rightly think or do,
Or make or spoil, or bless, or blast,
Is curse or blessing justly due
For sloth or effort in the past.
My life's a statement of the sum
Of vice indulged, or overcome.

As I wander on the roads
I shall be helped and healed and blessed;
Dear words shall cheer and be as goads
To urge to heights before unguessed.
My road shall be the road I made;
All that I gave will be repaid.

So shall I fight, so shall I tread,
In this long way beneath the stars;
So shall a glory wreathe my head,
So shall I faint and show the scars,
Until this case, this clogging mould
Be smithied all to kingly gold.

When Leslie Boyes came for healing he was feeling very low, but his wife says that, despite the serious illness — both mental and physical — he was suffering, he always went home afterwards happier and feeling better physically.

Four years on, Leslie had a stroke and after eight months in hospital, he died. I talked a lot with Denise after her husband's death, when she was feeling very distraught, lost and lonely. In time she found she was able to begin to understand things that had not been clear before. She sensed that her husband was still close by, and this was a great comfort to her.

The assumption that life begins at birth and ends at death, in the absence of evidence to the contrary, lays a particular importance upon the physical life – which would be grossly out of proportion if in fact that assumption was untrue. You and your body come together when you are born into this world – before that, they existed separately. YOU therefore existed before this life. Set against the 'fact' of your being, 'where' is almost irrelevant.

If you look upon the dead body of one you knew, it is clear that the body is no longer inhabited or animated by the person – we say that he or she is no longer there. We are aware that we are looking at what is only the body. So the person has merely separated from the body but has not ceased to be. As there is no beginning or end to time, there is equally no beginning or end to your being.

This begins to put our seventy or eighty years here into their proper perspective – our whole view of the value of material things begins to change with this understanding. Anything you think you own is in reality on loan and you only have the use of it for a while. You certainly can take none of it with you when you become separated from physical life. This lifts the burden of 'yours' and 'mine' and should increase the responsibility we have for whatever we are using.

An absent healing patient, writing from Seattle, quoted the following thought from Stuart Wilde: 'Money is like manure: if you leave it stacked up it just smells. But if you spread it around, it makes the flowers grow!'

As your adventure of 'being' never comes to an end, the prospect of the endless opportunity to learn stretches before you. As there is no signpost marked 'end of time' or 'end of being' there is no point in hurrying towards something which does not exist. It is therefore more intelligent to slow down and make good use of 'now' – because in reality it is always 'now'. There is much to be missed whilst travelling too fast and anything travelling too fast suffers stress.

Grief and tension had become a way of life for Sue Pearsall after her father died, following a harrowing struggle with cancer. She came to see me three months later, completely distraught and in tears. We talked about what it is like to lose someone we love, and I told her about the death of Phillip after his motorbike accident. When I saw her again six weeks later she was feeling very much stronger and more relaxed, with a renewed sense of purpose. She describes healing as a turning point in her life, helping her come to terms with the suffering and death of her father.

The question of where one goes after losing the use of the body is similar to asking how much love any one place can contain – it is a question which does not have a physically measurable answer and there is really no need to ask it. Three-dimensional measurements cannot be made of any abstract. Perhaps we live a life in this world many times as apparently different people, perhaps not. Either way, it does not alter the fact that you exist and always will.

Look up at the sky on a clear night and you will realize that out there, in every direction, there is no boundary – limitless space containing endless numbers of other 'grains of sand' like our own small planet. It will help bring much else into perspective.

In the long run, everyone gets to go home, I promise you.

ALL IS WELL
(After the original by Canon Henry Scott Holland
of St Paul's Cathedral)

> Death is nothing at all
> I have only slipped away into the next room
> I am I and you are you
> Whatever we were to each other
> That we still are

Call me by my old familiar name
Speak to me in the easy way which you always used
Put no difference into your tone

Wear no forced air of solemnity or sorrow

Laugh as we always laughed at the little jokes we enjoyed
    together
Play, smile, think of me, pray for me
Let my name be ever the household word that it always was
Let it be spoken without effect
Without the trace of a shadow on it

Life means all that it ever meant
It is the same as it ever was
There is absolute unbroken continuity

Why should I be out of mind because I am out of sight?
I am but waiting for you
For an interval
Somewhere very near
Just around the corner
All is well

8

Absent Healing

As you think you travel; and as you love you attract.
You are today where your thoughts have brought you;
you will be tomorrow where your thoughts take you . . .
You will become as small as your controlling desire;
as great as your dominant aspiration.

James Allen

The note from my receptionist read: 'You may recall that I spoke to you of Catherine, a friend of a friend. We asked you for absent healing – she had cancer of the cervix. She has written to say that the doctors have told her the tumour has disappeared! So she has avoided chemotherapy and a hysterectomy. She's now on hormone replacement therapy, eating well and gaining more energy daily.'

Healing is a matter of asking. On more than one occasion I have opened a letter from someone who thanks me for a successful absent healing. (Absent healing is carried out without the patient being present). I then discover, in the same pile of letters, the patient's very first letter to me – unopened until that moment – asking me for absent healing. Beneficial change has taken place, without my being aware of it, simply because someone has asked.

People write from all over the world, asking for absent healing. Distance is no barrier to the healing process and many are helped. Dealing with my correspondence, I first go through the letters I have received, one by one. I then write back to each person to confirm that I am seeking healing for the patient. I ask them to let me know when they find improvement. After that, I go through the letters again and ask the Guv'nor for healing for each individual. Many are kind enough to include a donation for my work which is always gratefully received, and helps towards expenses.

People sometimes feel an improvement in their condition without knowing that a friend or relative has asked for absent healing for them. A woman wrote asking for more details of absent healing (for her husband who was suffering from cancer). At the time of writing she was merely hoping for more information so was surprised to receive my reply saying that I was seeking healing for her husband and would be glad to know if he experienced any relief from his trouble. One month later the woman wrote back to say that her husband had started feeling better two days before she received my letter stating that healing had been sought. Her husband had not known anything about his wife's request until he read the reply from me.

Although I have found contact healing to be of greater benefit generally, there is no doubt that absent healing, too, can bring about wonderful changes both in a person's physical and mental state.

Neither distance nor the type or severity of the dis-ease makes any difference to the possibilities of absent healing. Patients often write back to let me know their progress: A man in his mid-sixties wrote from Victoria, Australia, telling me of the improvement in his spine. He had previously been suffering severe pain as a result of a degenerative condition. He had also been mourning the loss of his wife, and found that healing had been of great help and inspiration to him in his own spiritual journey.

A woman living in Indiana, USA, had fallen down a flight of steps and injured her back, ending up with two herniated discs and a pinched nerve. Doctors and a spell in hospital had done nothing to alleviate her pain and she was told that surgery was inadvisable. She wrote to tell me that she noticed a change the day she received my reply to her request for absent healing, and could now go for weeks without medication.

A man had brought his father back from his home in Greece in a very serious condition. A tumour had spread in his throat and he could no longer speak or even eat properly. A friend described the situation: 'He really was on his last legs – he only just made the distance from the airport terminal to the car. The family spent thousands of pounds, getting him back to England and admitted to the Royal Marsden Hospital. Doctors in Greece had said that there was nothing more they could do for him.' At the hospital she rang me and I asked her for the patient's name and a few other details. The next day the son went to visit his father. To his amazement he found him sitting up in bed, having pulled the drip off during the night. He was able to speak and eat again. Soon he was up and about and after two weeks, went back to Greece. In fact he did not have long to live, but his last days were free of pain and stress.

In Norway, a wheelchair-bound woman had suffered with a large, deep pressure sore in her back for one and a half years. Doctors had been unable to help. After absent healing the wound, as well as a urine infection, cleared up. And a woman in Natal, South Africa who had suffered for many years with chronic diarrhoea, mild fever and nausea, wrote: 'Strangely enough, the day you wrote to me I was very ill – terrible stomach ache, etc. By the time your letter arrived here, a week later, I was feeling much better and have not been ill since . . .'

There are some patients who fear they may not 'deserve' healing. Many letters contain the words 'I know how much worse off others are'. But I quickly reassure them that no religious faith is necessary, that the Guv'nor's love (and therefore healing) is for everyone. And as there is no limit to his love, it follows that there is no limit to what healing might achieve. One woman wrote 'I know that I am asking for a miracle, and I know that miracles do happen – the problem is that I don't believe I deserve one'. So she was delighted to be able to report later on an improvement in the sight of her right eye, which had been worrying her.

In healing, whether contact or absent – as with orthodox medicine – no permanent cure is ever certain. One absent healing patient who had been suffering with depression had at first noticed a positive change in her thinking and continued to report an improvement in her condition over the next few weeks. But a few months later she told me she was feeling low again, so that even writing a simple letter was taking a great effort of will.

I am hopeful that, with more research, we may better understand how healing works so that it will be more readily accepted as a natural part of life, and I am always pleased to hear from medical doctors who have benefited from it. A doctor in his late thirties wrote telling me of his thyroid problems, high cholesterol, a gall stone and poorly functioning kidneys. He had been feeling tired, lethargic, restless and depressed. Although he did not ask for absent healing, I nevertheless included him in my petition to the Guv'nor. The man wrote back later to tell me he was feeling much better, physically and mentally.

It is also heartening to hear from patients who have not only experienced improvement in their physical dis-ease, but also in their outlook. An absent healing patient from Wales wrote: 'It's definitely the age where more and more people are becoming enlightened . . . I came out of this (illness) more aware spiritually and learnt answers to a lot of questions. I realize that the more knowledge you attain, the more you have to learn. The more I learn the more I realize that, at the end of a lifetime, you have only just begun to understand.'

RULES FOR BEING HUMAN

As far as learning to be human goes, the following *Rules* could well be those given to us before we are born, to guide us through this life. The only problem is we have forgotten them.

1. You will receive a body. You may like it or hate it, but it will be yours for the entire period this time around.

2. You will learn lessons. You are enrolled in a full-time informal school called life. Each day in this school you will have the opportunity to learn lessons. You may like the lessons or think them irrelevant and stupid.

3. There are no mistakes, only lessons. Growth is a process of trial and error experimentation. The 'failed' experiments are as much a part of the process as the experiment which ultimately 'works'.

4. A lesson is repeated until it is learned. A lesson will be presented to you in various forms until you have learned it. When you have learned it, you can then go on to the next lesson.

5. Learning lessons does not end. There is no part of life that does not contain its lessons. If you are alive there are lessons to be learned.

6. 'There' is no better than 'Here'. When your 'There' has become 'Here', you will simply obtain another 'There' that again will look better than 'Here'.

7. Others are merely mirrors of you. You cannot love or hate something about another person unless it reflects to you something you love or hate about yourself. If you hurt someone else you are hurting yourself.

8. What you make of your life is up to you. You have all the resources and tools you need. What you do with them is up to you. The choice is yours.

9. Your answers lie inside you. The answers to life's questions lie inside you. All you need to do is look, listen and trust.

10. You will forget all this.

Anon.

9

Some Questions Answered

Go beyond reason to love
It is safe
It is the only safety.

In spite of the growing awareness and acceptance that there is a spiritual reality existing alongside the material, there is also still much doubt and even suspicion about healing. What people do not understand they often fear. Yet we all understand love – and love is what healing is really about. Quite simply, the power of love. Love has no limitations, which includes the love within each one of us. It follows therefore that there is no limit to what healing can achieve. People speak of the 'supernatural', but there is no such thing. 'Natural' can only ever be just that. 'Supernormal' is the term given to something outside our experience, but the supernormal is still within the whole, natural law.

Healing is not fortuitous or magic or miraculous. It is part of the natural law; part of the whole truth of our existence that we have not fully understood. Through this book it is hoped that the foundations for a greater understanding might be laid, a more open attitude that will lead to further investigation. Healing is part of life – why not explore it? We hear increasingly these days of the different approaches to healing – hypnosis, healing magnetism, 'spiritual' healing. And there is growing interest in alternative treatments such as herbal remedies and yoga for relaxation. But because we are all ONE, our health depends, largely, on the love around us, in our relationships with each other. That is why I refer simply to 'healing': the wonderful changes in both mind and body that are achieved by nothing more than the power of love.

Questions and doubts are often raised, on some of which I have given my own thoughts here.

Q: Do you ever go to a G.P. yourself?
A: Of course! And thank God for doctors. What's more, I always make a point of asking my patients what their own doctor has to say about their condition. Medicine is part of the Guv'nor's world, so why not? After all, I have a body and doctors specialize in the body so there is no reason why one should dispense with them. You have heard St Luke's words: 'Physician, heal thyself', but of course I do not heal anyone. Healing comes from the Loving Spirit.

Q: Will I have to pay?
A: We never ask for payment at Roundstreet and no invoice is ever sent. However, donations enable me to carry on with what I do! Healing is not a business in any way – the only one I work for is the Guv'nor. Donations, though, mean I can pay for such necessities as electricity, heating, telephone etc.

Q: What about healing for animals?
A: I do not deal with animals but there are healers who do – and some who give healing to both humans and animals.

Q: Why is it that there are not long queues at your door?
A: There *are* times when many people want to come for healing. But I deliberately try and avoid too busy a schedule. I make sure that each person who comes is given plenty of time to talk, so this will always limit the number of people I can see in a day. Sometimes my diary is fully booked for some weeks ahead but such things as holidays and the weather can make a difference. And of course people do have a habit of getting better! Another reason for the lack of queues is that people are still reluctant to tell others they have been to a healer, even if they get better. The thing is, healers are no different from anybody else and should never pretend to be. It would

be dangerous to let yourself be put on some sort of pedestal by trying to be something you are not – being human, you would be sure to fall off sooner or later!

Q: Do healing benefits ever wear off?
A: This is far less likely if the causes within the patient, as well as the resulting dis-ease in the body, are dealt with. The physical symptoms of an illness may be put right with a bottle of pills from the doctor, but there is never any guarantee that the condition will not reappear – particularly if the underlying cause has not been recognized. It is the same with healing.

John Pilkington suffered years of pain following a serious back injury. Healing was successful where all types of medical intervention had failed to help. But John's work involved a great deal of heavy lifting, and I warned him that until he was able to give up this type of work, his back would never heal completely. He still occasionally comes back for healing after he has overdone things and aggravated the injury again, but he has not had to go back to a doctor.

Q: If love is in us all, why is there so much trouble in the world?
A: An interviewer, watching Mother Theresa caring for a dying Indian beggar, asked 'How do you regard this man?' Her reply was 'I see him as God who happens to have caught a bit of a cold.' None of us is perfect – there is good and bad in each one of us. We need to look for the goodness (that is, 'God-ness') that exists in everyone. I believe goodness will win because the power that created the entire universe is love and everybody has that love within them. You might look at it this way: You can shine light into darkness and dispel it but you can never do it the other way round – white needs black in order to be visible. It is because of our imperfections that we do the damage. People cry 'If there is a God, why does he allow such things to happen?' I came across one answer to this which made a lot of sense: If he *did* put everything right overnight, first thing next morning we would start messing it up again! And then the opportunities to learn would be denied

us. That is why we are here, simply to learn. A one-sided coin
is no use to anyone.

Q: Why are so many established religions suspicious of healing?
A: Religions like to think that they have all the answers and
that they know better than every other religion. It is rather
awkward for them that healing does not depend in any way
on religion. At one time, if someone did not belong to any
particular sect but healing still occured in them, a religious
would, quite likely, have put it down to the work of the
Devil. In this way they were able to continue using the
familiar weapon of fear. In the 39 Articles of the Church
of England, printed in the front of its prayer book, there
is no mention of healing. The official dogma until recently
was that healing was something that could only happen in
the name of Christ, in a church. However, they have begun
to notice that healing is happening *outside* the churches and
have had to think again. The official line now is that it can
in fact happen outside churches, and is alright really! Having
condemned healing for so long, they are now quite anxious
to get in on the act!

The Catholic Church cites Lourdes as evidence that they
have, of course, always approved of healing – and yet the fact
is that until recently their followers were given stern warnings
to keep away from healers!

I see organized religions as attempts by man to organize
God. But the natural beauty of a rose, for example, tells me
He is pretty well organized already!

Helena, a bright 22-year-old who came for healing for back
pain, told me the following story: One day a rather bossy
and forthright friend of her mother's arrived on the doorstep
with the vicar and another man who was introduced as the
'church healer'. The friend announced to Helena 'You are
going to be healed!' As the vicar already seemed to have
one foot in the door, Helena and her mother felt they had to
invite the visitors in. The church healer felt it necessary to start
praying in a sing-song voice, crying 'Jesus will heal her' and

carrying on at some considerable length. The performance went on for so long that Helena and her mother began to get rather fed up, at which point he changed tack and began to chant 'If you believe in Jesus he will heal you'. Finally, in exasperation, her mother declared 'Of course, you do realize that my daughter is Jewish!' The little deputation left in some confusion and a great hurry. In fact, she is half-Jewish, on her father's side, but not in the least bothered either way. I mention this little story simply to illustrate the nonsense of the sectarian view. The final irony being of course that Christ himself was a Jew!

Miracles have never ceased to happen since Christ walked on earth 2,000 years ago. Christ, though, was more than just a healer. Healers only channel the power, but Christ was so much of an avatar that the healing actually came from him. Everyone has God within them because God is Love, but from time to time someone turns up on earth who has this Love within them to an extraordinary degree. We call this person an avatar: a God-filled man.

I sometimes think of the Guv'nor as a mountain, with all the religions of the world living round its base. The religions come and go, but the mountain is constant – and it can be climbed. Only by climbing the mountain can we really know and understand it. I heard Hell described as 'A place where God is not'. To my mind, this illustrates a total lack of understanding. If 'God is all and all is God', how can there be a place where God is not?

People need to be helped to their own understanding without being subjected to one particular dogma – and it is sad that this is often delivered as Truth to the impressionable minds of children. A patient wrote to let me know of the improvement in her health following absent healing. In her letter she says '. . . we had religion and the Bible forced upon us – even a Bible in the loo! It created conflicts because in those days we did not understand God at all. When you are four years old and your mother dies, you do not understand when told that God is love . . . .'

My son Toby came home from school one day and said,

'Daddy, I don't like our headmaster' (who happens to be a parson). I asked him why this was. 'Well,' Toby said, 'he makes us go to chapel every morning and when we are in there he tells us we have got to love one another and be nice to each other – but when we come out he is horrid to us all!'

Q: Do you ever refuse anyone?
A: Yes. I will not treat infectious diseases. And I would much rather people did not come to me with a streaming cold! Many do, surprisingly – perhaps they think I am immune! Sometimes it becomes obvious, over a period of time, that a patient is not going to respond to healing. This is the sort of person who is not prepared to listen, who simply wants attention and not healing. In a way, they want to hang on to their illness because of the notice and sympathy it brings. There is no point continuing when someone is wasting your time as well as their own.

Q: What about self-help – diet, exercise and meditation, etc?
A: Of course. We should all be responsible and do whatever we can to help ourselves. I would always advise people to look at their diet and read up about the subject. What you have to remember though is that you are not a machine. What is right for one person may not be right for another, because everyone is different. You have something wonderful inside you which is called instinct or intuition. We all know how a pregnant woman will sometimes eat the most astonishing things. This is simply her body telling her what she specifically needs. It is the use we make of what we eat that matters, rather than letting it make use of us.

Actually, I get fed up when 'experts' tell us what we should or should not do. We now have artificial salt and sugar. The real things, we are told, are bad for us. If that is really so, why aren't we all dead? We got along splendidly for years before the advent of the expert! A patient came to me with lung and throat cancer, hardly able to speak or breathe. He was sixty-six and had stopped smoking just before Christmas. The disease had started just after Christmas and doctors told him it was the stress and shock to his system of giving up smoking that had triggered it. Nicotine has been found harder to give up even than heroin. No-one should encourage smoking of course, but the sensible rule surely is: moderation in everything.

Q: What does healing offer that orthodox medicine does not?
A: Orthodox medicine deals mostly with the body. Even medicine that is supposed to deal with the mind – psychiatry – uses more drugs than any other sector of the medical profession. This means that in trying to treat the mind they are still only dealing with the body. Healing on the other hand deals with the whole person, not just the effects of an illness but its very source. Healing is a gentler art – it is only ever offered, never forced.

In fact, healing and orthodox medicine can often complement each other. Bad healers and charlatans have been responsible for the suspicion still felt by some doctors. The truth of what healing is really about needs to be known, so that there is no more suspicion or fear. The more sensible understanding there is of it, the less room there will be for the frauds – because people will know what healing actually involves and what to expect from a healer. As our knowledge improves, it will be accepted that there is such a thing as healing which is not simply spontaneous remission.

Q: What type of person comes to you? Are they usually 'believers' in what you do?
A: I see every type of person, from all different sectors of society. The success of healing does not depend upon blind faith, although a little faith may help. In fact some people who come are totally cynical. They are giving healing a try because their spouse or a friend has persuaded them that they ought to. Others have virtually given up hope of getting better and feel that, whatever happens, they have nothing to lose.

I also meet people who arrive full of religious fervour –

which does not of course guarantee healing in any way! People without any sort of faith receive healing just as often – young babies for instance: one-year-old Emily was brought by her mother with serious kidney problems that had been diagnosed before birth. Antibiotics had failed to clear up a urinary tract infection, and tests showed that both kidneys had scar tissue. The child was often in pain. After healing, Emily started to sleep through the night, then started to drink three times as much as she had previously. Four months later X-rays showed that the scar tissue had disappeared and she had considerably improved. Her mother regrets that she only decided to try healing as a last resort.

I do think that healing needs the co-operation of the patient as far as his or her willingness to accept its message is concerned. A young man came to me recently who told me he had been in prison. He was still in the habit of lying, cheating and stealing and I believe that this was the reason he did not get better. He was in fact a basically nice person, but was not prepared to give up his old ways of thinking and behaving.

There is something better than faith – and that is knowing. Believing is not knowing, whatever Christians might say. Believing is more subject to error than actual experience. When religions say 'You are not supposed to know', what they mean is that they themselves do not know. This is just as bad as the politician who has never been further than his own home town but who is quite happy to tell the rest of the world what it should be doing!

Q: Does having 'someone to listen' help the healing?
A: Yes, of course. We all benefit from the opportunity, in an atmosphere of openness and care, to speak from the heart. Mind you, I am a failed Samaritan! During our training we were asked to act out various situations that might arise in our work. One girl had to pretend to be pregnant and threatening suicide. I listened to her tale of woe then told her that she should start to think of her situation as something wonderful – the advent of human life into the world is a tremendous event. And as it is the Guv'nor who gives life, not us, perhaps

she could change her mind and realize what a splendid thing was happening to her. She should try not to worry too much about tomorrow but think about today.

Everyone, including the vicar who ran the group, was rather put out. I should apparently have talked about abortion instead. This is a suggestion I would never have made – being quite well aware that, had there been free abortions when I was conceived, I would probably not have entered the world as I am. In the end we could not agree and the outcome was inevitable – I was asked to leave.

Q: In a healing session, what does the patient feel?
A: You will have read earlier in the book about the many different reactions which may be experienced by patients. One patient, Dee Pilkington, found that healing meant more to her than relief from the chronic back pain that she had suffered since the birth of her children. She describes it as an 'emotional tonic' and says it made her realize that she had control over her own body – that we all have the power within ourselves to heal most of the things that ail us.

People are often moved to tears – and I keep a box of tissues handy for the purpose! I think the reason for this is that in healing you are brought closer to the source of your being, which is bound to be a moving experience.

Q: Perhaps healing should be available on the National Health Service?
A: That is where it may end up, but I hope not. I have always believed in personal responsibility and this does not seem to play a large part in the thinking of the NHS.

Q: Can you sense the spirit world?
A: I have never been involved in this way in my work, although it is a natural part of life, an awareness that some – such as mediums – have. Telepathy is very commonplace of course. In normal conversation thought passes from mind to mind. The means being employed happen to be voice and ears. But this often takes place between two people without

the use of their physical senses when they are separated by distance, especially when there is love between them.

Q: Why is there a stigma – why do we still doubt?
A: Because we live in a material and materialistic world. As we have to deal with the material world all the time this usually takes precedence over everything else. I sometimes think of it as a case of 'throwing the baby out with the bath water', the way people disregard what is essentially important.

Q: Do some complaints respond better than others?
A: No. Some healers will tell you that they have particular success with, for instance, back trouble. But I should think the reason for this is that there are simply more cases of back trouble than anything else, so it is the law of averages.

'I am afraid to come for healing. It all sounds a bit weird.'
Someone telephoned me one day and said 'Do you heal in the name of Christ?' I replied that I was not sure what she meant and began to ask her 'What about God?'. At which point she slammed down the telephone. I had no intention of being rude to her of course, but merely wanted to explain something about what I did. Yes, people do think it weird. The unfortunate thing is that some healers make it seem that way with all sorts of irrelevant rituals, chanting or whatever. The truth is that it could not be more simple or less weird. Healing speaks for itself.

'My doctor says it may do me more harm than good.'
The doctor of one of my patients did say just this, although the patient's condition improved dramatically after healing. I find that doctors who disapprove have either had no experience of healing or have had dealings with bad healers. A woman in her thirties came to see me once with a very advanced case of cancer. She had previously been to a group of healers on the south coast. These people had told her that they could only give her healing if she promised to dispense with all medical help! The poor woman was quite desperate with worry, not

knowing whether she should take this seriously or not. I was horrified. 'Healers' such as these are the ones who do the damage and make the medical profession understandably wary. The Roundstreet Healing Trust* hopes to make possible a better understanding of how healing may best be practised, through doctors' observation of it.

'It is probably a case of mind over matter.'
Isn't everything! The mind does come into everything. Healing in fact does not depend on the mind but it certainly helps to use your own mind rather than let something else use it. You can choose to think a positive thought, but you can also let a negative one in. Your body, for instance, is a product of what you eat – and this is an obvious case of mind over matter. 'All in the mind' does not mean that it is unreal, which is purely materialistic thinking. Because your mind is not made of material matter it is immensely flexible and subject to change – if YOU choose to change it. I always talk openly with my patients but I would never try to make them think as I do. This would only be encouraging them to make all the mistakes I myself continue to make! I simply tell my patients what I think and if they can make use of it, that's fine. If they don't want to, that's fine too. The sad thing is that there are so many people walking about who do not use their minds. Yes, mind over matter is very real.

'Everyone gets ill – it's normal. Old people have always had arthritis.'
Disease is the result of stress. By no means all my elderly patients come to me with arthritis – it's not compulsory as

---

* The Roundstreet Healing Trust has been set up with the aim of establishing a healing centre. This would provide a base for:

1. Research into healing, in conjunction with orthodox practitioners
2. Those requiring accommodation during an intensive course of treatment

It is also the aim of the trust, which is dependent on charitable donations, to subsidise treatment for those patients unable to meet the costs themselves.

you get older! But stress will find expression in one way or another. One splendid old lady (who eventually died aged ninety-six, simply from a 'surfeit of life') had come to me because she was suffering from depression. She in fact looked twenty years younger than she was, had a marvellous smile and was upright and charming. She was a sweet woman whom everyone adored. The only person who did not know how nice she was, was HER. We must be kinder to ourselves, or we will become ill from lack of care. I am glad to say that healing was successful in lifting the depression. Incidentally, this lady only had a very little arthritis, which did not bother her.

The truly wonderful thing about healing is that it is not simply about treating 'dis-ease'. Once you realize the implications of the power involved – and where it comes from – you know that nothing is impossible. You then have the marvellous knowledge that your own SELF has no limitations. Healing the 'kit' is just the beginning of the story. What it means and where that meaning takes us on our inward journey is the exciting part – for this is the beginning of our discovery of Truth.

Useful Addresses

If you would like to enquire personally for healing, please write (enclosing a stamped, addressed envelope) to:

Phil Edwardes
Roundstreet House
Wisborough Green
West Sussex RH14 OAN

Or just call 0403 700349 – Tuesday to Friday inclusive, after 10.00 a.m. and before 5.00 p.m.

For information about the Roundstreet Healing Trust (Registered Charity No. 328531) and its work, write to The Roundstreet Healing Trust at the above address enclosing a s.a.e.

National Federation of Spiritual Healers (NFSH)

Old Manor Farm Studio
Church Street
Sunbury-on-Thames
Middlesex TW16 6RG

Overseas Affiliates of the NFSH

Africa

Southern Africa Federation of Spiritual Healers
Mrs L E Jones
PO Box 501
Valyland 7978
Cape
Republic of South Africa Tel: 021 852320

The Healing Association of South Africa
Ms Katharine Lee-Kruger
The Leeward
6 El Corro Centre
130 Weltevreden Road
Northcliff Ext 6
Johannesburg
Republic of South Africa

America

National Federation of Spiritual Healers of America Inc
Rev Nancy Love (President)
PO Box 2022
Mount Pleasant
South Carolina
29465
America

Mr Charles Blackburn (Chairman)
9 W Walnut Street 1-D
Asheville
North Carolina
28801
America Tel: 010 1803 849 1529

Australia

Australian Spiritual Healers Association
PO Box 421
Gatton
Queensland 4343
Australia

Canada

National Federation of Spiritual Healers (Canada) Inc
Mrs Noreen Hodgson
T H 64/331 Military Trail
West Hill
Scarborough
Ontario
Canada
MIE 4E3 Tel: (416) 284 4798

Israel

Meditation for Peace and Harmony Group (MPH Group)
Mrs M Charney
17 Kerem Hazitim Street
PO Box 3380
Savyon
56540
Israel

New Zealand

New Zealand Federation of Spiritual Healers Inc
Ms R Younger
PO Box 9502
Newmarket
Auckland
New Zealand

* * *

The Doctor-Healer Network
19 Fore Street
Bishopsteignton
South Devon TQ14 9QR
Tel: 0626 779218

MUSIC IN THE MEMOIR

MUSIC PLAYS A FUNDAMENTAL ROLE in this story, certain pieces becoming virtual characters in the plot. If you are not familiar with some of the classical music mentioned in this memoir, I have included many of the works on my Author Page, www.JulieScolnik.com, with links to YouTube performances and recordings. I hope you will take a moment to listen.

1. Mozart: "Voi che Sapete" from *The Marriage of Figaro*
2. Berlioz: Judex crediris from Te deum
3. Ibert: *La berceuse du petit zébu*
4. Mahler: *Adagietto* from Symphony No. 5
5. Beethoven: *Adagio molto e cantabile* from Symphony No. 9
6. Brahms: *Andante* from Piano Quartet in C Minor
7. Rameau: *La nuit*
8. Mozart: "Bei Männern" from *The Magic Flute*
9. Jean Ferrat: *Ma France*
10. Schubert: *Andante* from Trio in B-flat
11. Liszt: *Au bord d'une source*
12. Michel Legrand: *The Umbrellas of Cherbourg*
13. Mozart: Requiem: Lacrimosa from Requiem in D Minor
14. Chopin: *Larghetto* from Piano Concerto No. 2
15. Beethoven: *Cavatina* from String Quartet Op. 130
16. Menotti: "Monica's Waltz" from *The Medium*

you gave me so many other chances? How could I not see that you couldn't let go any more easily than I could when you kept appearing unannounced at the chorus? The eyes from across the piano, one look amongst a hundred.

Then finally you did move on. You married, and you had your own children. And I have not been able to ask you a single question about this man you call your husband. You were not supposed to be with anyone but me. Why do you think I suddenly had no time for you in Boston when I learned you were pregnant with your son? Why do you think I didn't return your phone calls when you came to Paris with your daughter? Your charming, musical daughter—the very image of you. You were the love of my life and will always be the woman I was meant to be with, the one who saw into me, the mother of the musical children you didn't have with me.

Those were the words I needed to read to release that hidden and immutable heartache from my youth, lurking unseen for so long. I closed my laptop and went up to bed, Anya following close behind.

END